# Clinical Uses of Dreams in Psychoses

This groundbreaking work challenges traditional psychoanalytic practice by demonstrating how dreams can be effectively utilised in treating psychotic patients.

The book provides comprehensive solutions to clinical challenges faced when working with psychotic patients and their dreams. It addresses the difficulty patients experience in distinguishing between dreams, reality, and delusions, while tackling the problems some psychotic patients face with free association and the prevalence of disturbing nightmares. The work establishes how dreams fundamentally contribute to treatment by putting ineffable experiences into discourse, enabling historisation, and replacing traditional free association with dream chaining. The methodology emphasises careful interrogation of dreams through focused questioning that connects dream content to the patient's life and subjective position, ultimately allowing psychotic patients to review and modify their relationship with the unconscious.

This essential resource is designed for psychoanalysts, clinical psychologists, psychiatrists, and mental health professionals working with psychotic patients who seek practical, evidence-based approaches to incorporating dream work into their therapeutic practice.

**Dr. Celeste Labaronnie** is a clinical psychologist and researcher specializing in the treatment of psychoses. She holds a Ph.D. in Psychology from the National University of La Plata, Argentina. She serves as an international peer reviewer for scientific journals in Brazil, Colombia, Mexico, and Argentina. Since 2026, she is registered with the Australian Health Practitioner Regulation Agency (AHPRA) and practicing in Perth.

# Clinical Uses of Dreams in Psychoses

## A Psychoanalytic Approach

**Celeste Labaronnie**

**Translated by**
**Bruno Colantoni**

Routledge
Taylor & Francis Group
LONDON AND NEW YORK

First published 2027
by Routledge
4 Park Square, Milton Park, Abingdon, Oxon OX14 4RN

and by Routledge
605 Third Avenue, New York, NY 10158

*Routledge is an imprint of the Taylor & Francis Group, an informa business*



*British Library Cataloguing-in-Publication Data*
A catalogue record for this book is available from the British Library

ISBN: 978-1-041-27587-9 (hbk)
ISBN: 978-1-041-27591-6 (pbk)
ISBN: 978-1-003-75516-6 (ebk)

DOI: 10.4324/9781003755166

Typeset in Times New Roman
by Newgen Publishing UK

# Contents

# About the Author

Dr. Celeste Labaronnie is a clinical psychologist and researcher specializing in the treatment of psychoses. She holds a Ph.D. in Psychology and a specialization in Psychoanalytic Clinic from the Universidad Nacional de La Plata (UNLP), Argentina. Her extensive professional background includes serving as a Research Fellow for the Secretariat of Science and Technology at UNLP and teaching Psychotherapy at the university level.

In December 2025, her book *¿Cambian los sueños* a lo largo de *un análisis*? (2022) was awarded a Special Mention in the National Prize for Psychological Essay (Production 2019–2022) in Argentina. She has also authored *Usos clínicos de los sueños en las psicosis* (2019) and has published extensively in international peer-reviewed journals across France, Canada, the USA and Latin America.

Her professional experience spans over 17 years, including a clinical internship at the General Acute Care Hospital "Dr. Larrain". She serves as an international peer reviewer for scientific journals in Brazil, Colombia, Mexico, and Argentina.

Since 2025, she has been registered with the Australian Health Practitioner Regulation Agency (AHPRA), and she is currently practicing in Perth.

# Introduction

What do psychotics dream of? Do their dreams differ in any way from those of neurotics? Can it be of use to a psychoanalyst to listen to the dreams of their psychotic analysands? And if they do listen, will they authorise themselves to intervene? These questions broadly sketch the trajectory I follow in this book. The first set originates in psychiatry and was taken up by Freud at a very early stage; their earliest traces can even be found in philosophers and artists. The second, by contrast, belongs exclusively to psychoanalysis, and plunges into the heart of the analysis of psychotics, exploring there the potentialities of the dream.

The practice of interpretation as such, and of the interpretation of dreams in particular, was discouraged in the treatment of psychosis for many years – at least in certain sectors or generations of analysts. This may have been more a matter of corridor rumour than any properly documented contraindication, yet even today we witness the unease it provokes.

The theorisation of the analysis of psychotics has, however, advanced considerably in recent years, above all in the direction of reducing the prejudices that bore down upon it and lifting the encumbrances that at times made such analyses something of a second-hand practice – one of low expectations and little ambition.

A good number of works, published from various parts of the world, have cultivated the ground upon which the questions concerning the role of the dream in treatments with psychotics can today be raised in earnest. The topic has already been the object of meticulous and well-grounded elaborations – albeit scarce ones.

DOI: 10.4324/9781003755166-1

Our aim is to take up those works at their most clinical, setting aside certain theoretical paths that exceed our ambitions – in some cases, highly refined metapsychological debates – and to focus on the general lines of the theory that underpins some genuinely valuable clinical examples.

The first part of this book is largely phenomenological and includes some basic clinical clarifications. We begin from an ordering proposed by Freud for the works which, up to his time, had centred on the theme of dreams and mental diseases. There we explore the temporal relations between the psychotic episode and the dream, the analogies that classical psychiatry found between dream-work and the work of psychosis, and the particularities that florid psychosis induces in oneiric life and in the account of dreams in the session.

In the second part, we enter into the question of dreams in psychoses[1] in transference. We approach the theme guided by Freud, with his distinction between *verwerfung* and *verdrängung*, and then survey some of Lacan's ideas that return to the problem of the unconscious in the psychoses. We go on to address briefly the question of the rejection of the unconscious and its possible modalisations in analysis, giving priority to the proposals of analysts who advocate recognising the modifications that this position can undergo through the transferential encounter.

This ground allows us to advance upon the elaborations that have addressed the specific question of dreams in the analysis of psychotics and to delineate their central ideas. There we also articulate a proposal by Lacan concerning the relation between *jouissance* and language, which we find useful for thinking about dream-work and its effects.

We then go on to present two cases of psychosis reported by analysts in France and Canada, in which dreams form a central part of the analysis, of its progress, and of the subsequent account. We include some examples from our own clinical practice at the end of Section 6.3 and develop a case at length in Chapter 9. This is the Case of C., a patient seen at the Health Service of the National University of La Plata, as part of the clinical training for the Postgraduate Specialisation in Psychoanalytic Clinical Practice with Adults.

Finally, in Chapter 10, we gather together several observations concerning the technical and theoretical dimensions of working with dreams in the analysis of psychotic patients, drawing on the cases reported throughout the book.

## Note

1 Throughout this book, the term ‘psychoses’ is used in the plural wherever possible, in order to emphasise the wide variety of presentations this clinical structure encompasses and the fact that singularity seems even more pronounced within it than in the neuroses.

# Part 1

# Variants of the Dream-Psychosis Relationship

The possible relationships between dreams and psychosis are quite extensive; they can include the similarities that the clinician will find between the phenomena observed in psychotic episodes and dreaming, or the way in which dreams affect or are affected by periods of crisis.

This topic has already been addressed by Freud, who dedicated a complete section of "The Interpretation of Dreams" titled "The Relations between Dreams and Mental Diseases". Setting aside the fact that he refers to psychosis as an illness, we can find significant points in that section about the articulation of dreams with periods of psychotic episodes. There, Freud organises these relationships according to three axes:

> When we speak of the relation of dreams to mental disorders we may have three things in mind: (1) aetiological and clinical connections, as when a dream represents a psychotic state, or introduces it, or is left over from it; (2) modifications to which dream-life is subject in cases of mental disease; and (3) intrinsic connections between dreams and psychoses, analogies pointing to their being essentially akin.
>
> (Freud, 1900/1971, p.88)

We will follow this same organisation in order to present some ideas about each point. We will use examples provided by Freud and by the physicians of his time, some clinical descriptions from the DSM-IV, the *Memoirs* of Daniel Paul Schreber (1903/2000), Lacan's doctoral thesis (1932), and some of his comments found at different moments of his teaching.

DOI: 10.4324/9781003755166-2

# 1 Aetiological and Clinical Connections between Dreams and Psychosis

As we have seen, Freud identifies at least three possibilities here: that dream-life represents the psychotic state, that it introduces it, or that it is left over from it. Let us examine each case separately.

## 1.1 Psychotic Episodes Confined to Dream-Life

Dealing with patients whose psychotic episode remains entirely confined to dream-life does not seem to be common in psychoanalytic practice and is not frequently reported as part of the case studies on psychosis. However, Freud gathered interesting examples in his review of medical texts. He first comments on a state described by Allison (cited in Freud, 1900/1971), characterised by the appearance of hallucinatory phenomena and fits of rage at night in individuals who appear healthy during the day. This condition was named *nocturnal insanity*. As indicated by Freud, similar cases had been described by De Sanctis and Tissié.

Currently, the DSM-IV (1994) includes similar conditions in the section on *Parasomnias*, which are characterised by "abnormal behavioural or physiological events occurring in association with sleep, specific sleep stages, or sleep-wake transitions" (p.551). Among the parasomnias, the manual includes *Nightmare Disorder*, *Sleep Terror Disorder*, and *Sleepwalking Disorder*.

We are particularly interested in *Sleep Terror Disorder*, which, unlike *Nightmare* and *Sleepwalking Disorders*, involves an abrupt awakening that is not followed by a quick return to a state of wakefulness and orientation. Instead, the individual remains terrified for a period of time after partially waking up and screaming. The DSM-IV

DOI: 10.4324/9781003755166-3

specifies that the patient does not respond to others' efforts to comfort them, as they remain in a very particular state, which also entails total amnesia of the episode afterwards.

Of the states described by the manual, this one appears to be the most similar to the episodes of *nocturnal insanity* reported during Freud's time. What Allison observed fits very well with the current description of sleep terrors, although he is perhaps more categorical, as the panicky screams mentioned by the DSM are referred to by him as fits of frenzy, and the individual's continued immersion in the dream and difficulty waking – even when sitting up and surrounded by people – would seem to correspond to what Allison did not hesitate to classify as *hallucinations*. Despite this distinction, the difference between these classical descriptions and that of the DSM-IV seems to be more terminological in nature.

That said, we must specify that these conditions do not necessarily coincide with what we structurally consider psychosis in psychoanalysis. Nevertheless, they hold some interest for us due to the relationship they establish between dreams and waking life, where precisely what is observed is that these two states are not clearly separated for those who experience them. This is characteristic of many of the psychoses we encounter as analysts. Although we can say that dreams reveal our radical reality and that the Other scene is not independent of the scene of reality –which Lacan did not hesitate to put in continuity with the fantasy – we must specify that the difficulty in differentiating dream images from waking ones – at least those belonging to the present – is not common in neurotics and, instead, is part of the clinical picture of many psychoses. We will return to this topic in Section 2.1.

## 1.2 Dreams as Leftovers from Psychotic Episodes

At the beginning of Chapter IV of his *Memoirs*, D.P. Schreber explains that he suffered from nervous illness twice. The first time was during his candidature for parliament; the second was when he took up office as President of the Senate of a Court of Appeal in Dresden. In the interval between these two occurrences, he had dreams that he acknowledges as something left over from that first period.

> After recovering from my first illness I spent eight years with my wife, on the whole quite happy ones [...]. In June 1893 I was informed [...] of my impending appointment as *Senatspräsident*

> to the Superior Court in Dresden. During this time I had several dreams to which I did not then attribute any particular significance, and which I would even today disregard as the proverb says 'Dreams are mere shadows', had my experience in the meantime not made me think of the *possibility* at least of their being connected with the contact which had been made with me by divine nerves. I dreamt several times that my former nervous illness had returned; naturally I was as unhappy about this in the dream, as I felt happy on waking that it had only been a dream.
>
> (Schreber, 1903/2000, p.46; italics in original)

Many years later, having recovered from that second crisis, and retaining only a few delusional elements with which he managed quite well, Schreber explains that he also retained some dreams that were left over from that turbulent period:

> It is true that in the first years of my contact with God some information was imparted to me (partly in words, partly in the form of visions) apparently serving as instruction [...]. For some years such didactic communications have almost completely ceased; only very occasionally are there vision-like events in dreams which give the impression of a purposeful instruction. But I can not decide whether this is actually the case or whether it is only due to my nerves playing on me.
>
> (Schreber, 1903/2000, p.304, fn.120)

As we see, a certain type of dream, especially those that lead him to believe in divine influence, comes back to him from time to time. However, since he does not decide whether to attribute them the character of heteronomous revelations or mere "nerves playing" on him, the event has no major consequences; it remains circumscribed to dream-life. This circumstance corresponds to what Freud pointed out: "In cases of recovery from mental diseases it can often be quite clearly observed that, while functioning is normal during the day, dream-life is still under the influence of the psychosis" (Freud, 1900/1971, p.89).

However, it is worth noting that the expression "while functioning is normal during the day" calls for some reservations. On the one hand, because in psychoanalysis we do not draw a distinction between normal and abnormal[1]; and on the other, because the interpretive phenomena characteristic of psychosis may persist in individuals whom society might consider "recovered from their psychosis". Such was the case with Schreber, who had emerged from the acute phase of the crisis but still believed that his dreams could be the result of a divine influence – to name just one of the after-effects that he so richly described in his memoirs.

According to the information Freud extracts from the medical literature of his time, there were also cases described in which only in dreams did the patient relive the flight of ideas they had experienced during the psychotic episode, or at least some of the wild impulses that had invaded them at that time.

Many years later, Freud (1922/1981) reported two cases of paranoia that he treated, in which he was able to learn about the dreams that were occurring. In one of the cases, the dreams from the period after the psychotic episode were free of delusions. We will see later the details he extracts from there.

## 1.3 Dreams that Introduce Psychotic Episodes

Let us return to the paragraph from Schreber's *Memoirs* quoted earlier and see how it continues.

> After recovering from my first illness [...] I dreamt several times that my former nervous illness had returned; naturally I was as unhappy about this in the dream, as I felt happy on waking that it had only been a dream. Furthermore, one morning while still in bed (whether still half asleep or already awake I cannot remember), I had a feeling which, thinking about it later when fully awake, struck me as highly peculiar. It was the idea that it really must be rather pleasant to be a woman succumbing to intercourse. This idea was so foreign to my whole nature that I may say I would have rejected it with indignation if fully awake.
>
> (Schreber, 1903/2000, p.46)

We could say that the dreams Schreber had during that period between the first and second crises not only recalled the initial episode but also foreshadowed the subsequent one. These dreams occur while Schreber is in a very particular state. In fact, it is during this time that he experiences what Freud mentions as the *fantasy that appeared while he was half asleep* (Freud, 1911/1981, p.20).

What did the appearance of this fantasy while half asleep imply? Schreber points out that, had he been fully awake, he would have rejected it with indignation. It can be inferred from his statements, as well as from the *Memoirs* as a whole, that while in this state of being half asleep, he did not, in fact, reject this fantasy, but rather allowed it to take place. "[...] one morning, while still in bed (whether still half asleep or already awake I cannot remember)", he says, and explains that he reflected on this idea later, when he was fully awake, and that it then struck him in a very particular way. In short, his relationship with this thought that occurred in a state of being half asleep runs through all subsequent events described in the *Memoirs*: he struggles against this idea, partially accepts it, assumes it is imposed, combats it, but ultimately finds solace by granting it a place in his understanding of the universe.

With the genius that characterises him, Freud had observed that the relationship established by psychiatry between this type of oneiric thoughts and the subsequent pathological state warranted a revision in the light of his discoveries about the mechanisms of dreams and psychical life in general.

In 1830, Hohnbaum asserted that the outbreak of madness is often consequent upon an anxious or terrifying dream, and that even within it the central idea dominating the subsequent pathological condition can already be found (cited in Freud, 1900/1971). Similarly, other physicians argued that sometimes dreams are *the true determining cause of insanity* (Sante de Sanctis, cited in Freud, 1900/1971) – dreams that contain the delusional illumination and cause the psychosis to come to life at a single blow. In other cases, the possibility was also conceived that the delusional idea would develop slowly through a series of dreams (Freud, 1900/1971, p.88).

In this context, Freud speaks – paraphrasing the psychiatrists – of an "operative dream" (p.88) to refer to the one that brings to life the pathological state. However, he does not refrain from introducing a key distinction:

> In these instances the dreams are represented as the aetiology of the mental disorder; but we should be doing equal justice to the facts if we said that the mental disorder made its first appearance in dream-life, that it first broke through in a dream.
>
> (Freud, 1900/1971, p.89)

That is to say, the precedence of certain dreams regarding the subsequent episode does not necessarily imply a causal relationship, but rather a community of mechanisms, a delusional (paranoia) or dissociative (schizophrenia) state that will be expressed both through dreams and other phenomena. In this sense, the relationship between dreams and psychosis has been taken up in psychoanalysis, concerning the possibility of announcing an episode. Juan Pablo De Arriba, for example, speaks of dreams as an "index of destabilisation" (2018, p.198). The dream, when it occurs, is not a cause but rather another manifestation of the delusional or alienating ideas that begin to populate psychotic thinking at these critical moments. Nevertheless, this fact is of utmost interest to the clinician, and it is very common to hear that analysts become aware of the proximity of a psychotic episode when a known patient recounts certain types of dreams.

In his own way, Schreber explains this through the malleability of dreams to certain influences. What seems to him capable of invading waking life only under certain conditions, instead becomes a skilful usurper of dream-life:

> The rays therefore have the power to influence the nervous system and particularly the sensory nerves of a sleeping human being, in certain circumstances perhaps even those of a human being who is awake, in such a way that the person concerned thinks he can see strangers standing before him or hear them speak.
>
> (Schreber, 2000, p.73, fn.37)

Freud and Schreber agree, then, that the trigger of psychosis is not an operative dream; rather, a dream can sometimes be the first manifestation of an incipient episode – or the first demonstration of the impending divine influence, according to the latter.

Regarding the case of Schreber, Lacan precisely speaks of a "first dream of psychotic invasion" (Lacan, 1955–56/1997, p.256), taking the dream as the scene where the psychotic episode is announced before invading the patient's everyday life.

Sauvagnat & Sauvagnat (1998) have also focused on an example recounted by Lacan, involving one of his analysands. Apparently, this patient left him very concerned after recounting a certain dream, in which these authors locate the difficulty "in stopping the signifying chain" (p.459). The case is as follows:

> there is one of my patients – long ago, so that she will no longer hear this spoken of, otherwise I would not tell her story – one day she dreamed, just like that, that existence would always spring forth again by itself, the Pascalian dream, an infinity of lives succeeding one another endlessly; she woke up almost mad. She told me about it {laughter from the audience}. I, of course, did not find it amusing.
>
> (Lacan, 1972, p.7)

This dream once again puts us on the trail of Freud's question about the possible efficacy of dreams in precipitating a psychotic episode. We believe it is consistent to affirm that the concern Lacan refers to does not lie in any efficacy of the dream itself, but in the unsettling nature of something that is already happening, and that the dream, so to speak, shows, denounces, brings to the scene in advance: in this case, a continuity that could lead to madness. Sauvagnat & Sauvagnat (1998) comment: "It concerns a patient who dreams that death no longer exists. It seems evident that Lacan's concern regarding her has to do with the threat of a manic or melancholic episode" (p.459).

We conclude, then, that for psychoanalysts, dreams can serve as a warning of an impending psychotic episode. In this way, dreams often emerge as the initial manifestation of an impending crisis, with the dream scene being highly receptive to the subtle subjective changes that occur between the stages of crisis and stabilisation in certain psychoses.

## Note

1 Nor do we distinguish between the "healthy" and the "ill". At most, we may speak of a "surplus of suffering" that analysis can reduce, but we embrace no ideals of health, nor do we treat discontent in civilisation itself as a form of illness.

# 2 Alterations in Dream-Life in the Case of Mental Disease

Does the onset of a psychotic episode also affect dream-work? This could be said to be the underlying question behind several observations made by Freud regarding the relationship between dreams and psychosis. We will state from the outset what his answer will be: dream-work does not differ between neurosis and psychosis, not even during the acute phase of the psychotic episode. However, the way in which the patient may report their dreams, and especially how they interpret them, is indeed significantly affected by florid psychosis. What does not vary are the underlying mechanisms, which, as we will elaborate in Chapter 3, are common to both dreams and psychosis.

## 2.1 Continuity

We will first focus on how the dreamer reports their dream, how they recount it. Can marks of psychosis be found in the *way* a dream is recounted? Without hesitation: yes.

Psychotic patients sometimes move from recounting a dream to describing their current situation as if there were no discontinuity between the two. We should not assume that this will be a general feature in every psychosis, but when it does occur it is a valuable diagnostic element. Similarly, the form of the narration can reveal structural information when the account of the dream becomes disorganised, serving as a site for metonymic phrases, neologisms, or delusional assertions. In this respect, of course, the narration of a dream is no different from anything else the psychotic patient might wish to mention during the session. During acute episodes, it is quite common for us to be unable to distinguish whether what the patient

DOI: 10.4324/9781003755166-4

is attempting to recount is a dream, an event, an idea, or something else entirely.

But let us focus for now on this specific point: the experiential continuity that the psychotic may experience, at certain moments, between dream and waking life will result in a discursive continuity when recounting events in a session. In his account of the Case of Aimée – the paranoid patient to whom he dedicated his doctoral thesis – Lacan (1932) precisely highlighted this phenomenon:

> States of oneiric anxiety play an important role. In her dreams, the patient sees her son 'drowned, murdered, abducted by the G.P.U'. When she wakes, she is in a state of extreme anxiety. She is genuinely expecting, at any moment, the telegram informing her that the disaster has already occurred.
>
> (p.88)

Similarly, Schreber reported that during the psychotic episode it was impossible for him to determine whether certain events had been part of a dream or waking experiences. He writes, for instance:

> On [...] the night of the 14th to the 15th of March 1900/1971, there was wild play with miracles in my dreams, such as I had only experienced earlier (...). I eventually made an end to these wild miracles severely and anxiously disturbing my sleep, by forcing myself to wake up completely and turning on the light. It was only 11:30 p.m. (the door which leads from my room to the corridor was locked, so that nobody could have come in from outside). Despite this early hour of the night I immediately wrote it down on paper [...]. From the content of these notes I will here only quote that according to the vision produced by miracle in my dream, an attendant of the Asylum, whom I had first heard opening the door of the living-room adjoining my bedroom, was partly sitting on my bed, partly getting up to some mischief near my bed [...]; that I saw myself still in the dream vision having left the bed in order to turn on the light so that the miraculous visions should cease; but when I awoke fully I found myself still lying in bed so that I had not really left my bed at all.
>
> (Schreber, p.71, n.37)

In this account, we find two noteworthy characteristics. One is the dreamer's interpretation regarding the origin of his dream: the dream images were miraculously produced for him; it is not clear who the agent would be here, a matter he discusses in various sections of his book, without coming to definitive conclusions. The second is that he reports waking up within the dream: he believes he has woken up, but then realises that the subsequent experiences were also part of a dream. The latter is not surprising and is common in the phenomenology of dreams, but the former is pathognomonic of psychoses: thoughts, whether oneiric or not, are instilled in him. We will revisit this in Chapter 5.

We have mentioned the existence of cases where the psychotic episodes are confined to the night or to the state of sleep or being half asleep. Reviewing these cases has led us to the problem of the lack of differentiation between dreams and waking life, which is very common at certain moments of psychotic episodes. It is very interesting to pause and reflect on how Schreber ponders this issue:

> It is almost superfluous to waste words about such a common phenomenon as that a restlessly sleeping human being believes he sees dream visions which are conjured up, as it were, by his own nerves. But the dreams visions of the night just mentioned and similar earlier visions surpassed in their plasticity and photographic accuracy everything I had ever experienced when I was well. This cannot have been caused spontaneously by my own nerves, but must have been thrown into them by rays. [...] every other human being, had he seen similar dream visions, would equally have thought them real.
>
> (pp.72–73, n.37)

As can be seen, the dreamer considers that the inability to distinguish between dream visions and waking visions could be due to the difference between two conditions that he supposes: the personal origin of some images versus the imposed origin of others. If they were ordinary dream visions, he argues, they would not have the plasticity and photographic accuracy they have in his memory, which leads him to believe that they are imposed images.

If we continue to pay attention to the difficulty of distinguishing between dream and hallucination reported by Schreber, we can appreciate that, in his *Memoirs*, this issue has forced him to make several reformulations, which he has particularly placed in the footnotes.

> Naturally I have to modify some of my earlier statements [...]; in particular I can no longer doubt but that my meeting our reigning King, an account of which is given in footnote 28, was only a dream vision. In what follows I will therefore only touch on similar dream visions which I had without number in the early years of my illness; I will concentrate mainly on those events during which I am certain that I was in a waking state.
>
> (Schreber, 1903/2000, p.73, n.37)

These corrections, which he introduces to diminish the reality of events he previously believed he had experienced, reveal his difficulty in separating what he saw in waking states (hallucinatory or not) from what he saw while asleep. This difficulty is evident in his case to the extent that, tired of such imprecision, he decides to report only what he is certain he experienced. However, later on, he encounters doubts again. Now he faces the opposite case: what he was convinced was a dream may have been experienced while awake, in the form of a hallucination.

> Although in footnote 37 above I remarked that I no longer doubted that this was only a dream vision, I must again on further consideration restrict this view. That I was standing by the peep-hole of my bedroom door is too distinct a recollection to attribute to a hallucination. I would, however, concede the possibility that what I presumed to have seen outside the door could have been a hallucination (compare Kraepelin as quoted at the end of this chapter).
>
> (Schreber, 1903/2000, p.80 n.39)

We see that his doubts revolve around dream, waking life, and hallucination. Schreber reconsiders the status of these memories each time he recounts them. As Lacan (1932) commented regarding Aimée, "the affective states of sleep blend with daytime persecutions" (p.85).

From a psychoanalytic perspective, it could be added that this indistinction between dream and waking life admits many variations, and the analyst often perceives the situation through subtleties in language use. Some psychotic patients, for example, express that they are going to recount a dream, without expressing doubts about its oneiric nature. However, during the narration, they switch from past tense to present tense, leaving the analyst perplexed as to whether what is being narrated is, then, something that is currently happening. The continuation of a narrative in the transferential scene – one that initially purported to be a description of oneiric images – is one of the subtleties that the analyst's ear discerns with finesse.

Another of these subtleties is the truly palpable affectation of the patient who, being ready to recount a dream, and perhaps without incurring modifications of verb tenses, is so shaken by the narrative as if they were experiencing it in the present. Here we encounter another type of dream-waking life continuity, a continuity of affect, of affectation.

We can therefore conclude that the condition of *nocturnal insanity* reported by Freud from the medical literature, along with the *sleep terrors* described in the DSM-IV, are insufficient to characterise what we find in the analysis of psychotic patients: namely, a continuity between dream and waking life which, in our view, deserves to be placed at the centre of our observations on the relationships between dreams and psychosis. Our clinical and diagnostic judgements thus give more weight to this continuity – almost never observed in cases of neurosis – than to the relatively infrequent fact that psychotic episodes may be considered confined to the night or to dreams.

To these clarifications about the relationship of origin between dreams and psychotic episodes, we must also add the common occurrence in which a certain dream, or a particular relationship with dreams, defines the diagnosis of psychosis in transference for the analyst. This includes Schreber's delusional interpretations concerning the heteronomous origin of his dreams, but also certain types of dreams reported by analysts, in which the impossibility of establishing a cut, stopping, or setting limits is manifested and defines the diagnosis.

In the case of C., we will see that her recurring dreams exhibited this quality, unusual in neurosis, of unfolding the fall into the void as a scene capable of inhabiting time, rather than being confined to a brief gap between dream and awakening as is usually the case with this type of dream in neurosis. Another form of continuity puts us on the trail of psychosis here: the continuity of existence of an uninhabitable space such as the fall into the void.

## 2.2 The Interpretation

As we saw earlier, Schreber insists in his *Memoirs* on the heteronomous origin of his dreams: the dream images are instilled in him, divine rays send him those thoughts, his dreams are actually miraculous messages, divine illuminations that do not stem from his dream activity, but from a higher being, which places them in him. We see in this that the way the psychotic analysand interprets their dreams can be one of the clearest diagnostic data for the clinician. This does not mean that the psychotic subject cannot, once the transference is established and after certain advances in the treatment, appropriate their dreams and extract from them information about their singular way of elaborating their subjective crises and the symptoms that afflict them. But at the beginning of the treatment, it often happens that some psychotics report their dreams as coming from external forces and attribute to them a function in the scene of delusion.

> In my case, however, since my nervous illness took the above-mentioned critical turn, my nerves have been set in motion *from without* incessantly and without any respite. Divine rays above all have the power of influencing the nerves of a human being in this manner; by this means God has always been able to infuse dreams into a sleeping human being.
>
> (Schreber, p.55; italics in original)

The relationship between the psychotic dreamer and their dreams was particularly considered by Freud (1922/1981) in his report on two cases of paranoia. One of his patients showed a healthy scepticism towards his paranoiac fantasies and, consequently, also dismissed the dreams that took them as material. This aspect deserves to be highlighted, as it constitutes an exceptional condition for possible work with dreams in cases of psychosis – one in which a distance between the subject and the phenomena is already established, allowing him to go on to interrogate his productions.

When this does not occur, that is, when this distance between the dreamer and their dreams has not been established, then the circumstance arises in which the psychotic takes ideas from the dream material and connects them to various elements of the delusion. In this sense, in his thesis, Lacan mentions dreams as one of the materials – alongside the delusion itself and common perceptions – from which the psychotic patient, during the period of destabilisation, can extract ideas that end up being transformed into memory-images, illusions of memory in whose actual occurrence they will believe. He says regarding Aimée:

> Thus, the phenomenon was reduced to an illusion of memory. [...] These disturbances consist solely in an insufficiency of recollection, which allows a phantasmatic image (itself evoked by the associations of a perception, a dream, or a delusional complex) to be transformed into a memory-image.
>
> (Lacan, 1932, p.127)

As we will see in Chapter 6, a group of Canadian analysts, who have been working with dreams in treatments with psychotic patients, have clearly reported this issue. They point out that, initially, it is common for dreams to emerge in the treatment in continuity with delusion and not be differentiated from it, but if the treatment progresses, at some point dreams begin to be produced that serve other purposes, which even become central for the psychotic in order to historicise, recognise their subjective position, and question it.

In this section, we have been led from the position of interpreter of the psychotic, who often attributes their dreams to the effect of an external influence, to the material from which the dream is formed, that is, the thoughts that underlie it – delusional or not – which allows us to move on to the next point.

## 2.3 Dream-Thoughts

This is the third point we are interested in mentioning regarding the alterations that occur in dream-life during psychotic crises: the one concerning the material with which those dreams are formed, that is, the preconscious thoughts that underlie them, which may also present certain peculiarities, as they may themselves be delusional or fragmented thoughts. These thoughts will then be worked on by the dream by means of the usual mechanisms, but the final product will reveal the elementary phenomena upon which they have been constructed.

Freud (1922/1981) dedicated several paragraphs to this issue in his article on the mechanisms common to jealousy, paranoia, and homosexuality. As we mentioned, there he reports some observations on the treatment of two paranoiac patients. The first exhibited marked delusional jealousy; the second suffered from persecutory paranoia. "My two cases of paranoia showed an instructive contrast in the behaviour of their dreams", he explains (Freud, 1922/1981, p.229). Regarding one of these cases, he writes the following:

> The dreams of my jealous patient presented me with a great surprise. They were not simultaneous with the outbreaks of the attacks, it is true, but they occurred within the period which was under the dominance of the delusion; yet they were completely free from delusion and they revealed the underlying homosexual impulses with *no more than the usual degree of disguise*. Since I had had little experience of the dreams of paranoics, it seemed plausible at the time to suppose that it was true in general that paranoia does not penetrate into dreams.
>
> (Freud, 1922/1981, p.227; italics added)

Two things should be emphasised from this paragraph. First, Freud's confirmation that the mechanisms of dreaming and their distortion did not, in this case, exhibit characteristics different from those he knew from his analyses of neurotics; the degree of disguise was no greater than usual. Second, this patient's dreams were devoid of delusion, implying that the preconscious thoughts that his dreams took up and reworked were not originally delusional thoughts.

Freud's initial belief that paranoia does not penetrate into dreams would later be contradicted by what he observed in the second patient:

> Whereas those of the first case were free from delusion, as has already been said, the other patient produced great numbers of persecutory dreams, which may be regarded as forerunners of or substitutes for the delusional ideas. The pursuer, whom he only managed to escape with great fear, was usually a powerful bull or some other male symbol which even in the dream itself he sometimes recognized as representing his father.
>
> (Freud, 1922/1981, p.229)

In our view, it is very likely that we are here facing dream content that should not be hastily labelled as originating from delusion. In part it does, insofar as it corresponds to a dream elaboration of a persecutory concern that the patient also presented while awake. We must note, however, that it is not a dream that the patient interprets as revealing a delusional truth previously unknown to him; nor does it lead him to confuse the scenes of dream and waking life. Rather, it presents a concern similar to what a neurotic brings to analysis – one that often penetrates into dreams and is confessed through working with them. Only the delusional insistence on the original idea allows Freud to establish a link between dream and psychosis in this case. However, we must emphasise that this idea is no more delusional than any neurotic concern, and that the central point in this case is that it does not induce in the patient the certainty of some dark will of the Other operating in his dream.

Nevertheless, Freud's observation is interesting and instructive for a whole series of cases where the preconscious ideas that the dream utilises are indeed markedly delusional, or reveal the features of disorganisation and fragmentation characteristic of schizophrenia.

During our residency at a public hospital, we heard from a psychotic patient dreams in which parasites emerged from her vagina, along with other dreams of a similar nature, in which a delicate back-and-forth between delusional interpretation and bodily fragmentation appeared to constitute the preconscious material upon which the dream constructed its linguistic elaboration. These dreams – particularly due to their rawness and their lack of veiling – can be taken as an example of how, during florid psychosis, the dream does not differ in its mechanisms but does differ in the type of material it draws from the preconscious.

In schizophrenia, we will find that the material the dream works with may come from hallucinations or ideas corresponding to what Freud termed "organ-speech" (1915/2000b, p.198), all of which are subsidiary to the phenomena of bodily disintegration inherent to schizophrenia, or from phenomena of thought echo and thought disorganisation, which may pass into the dream as prior ideas or experiences and be reworked by its operation, being inserted into some narrative.

In Section 4.1, we will see that the comments Freud introduces in the aforementioned text on the two cases of paranoia are valuable for thinking about the usefulness of dreams in analysis with psychotic patients, insofar as they point to this quality of dream-work: its capacity to gather and disguise – also in psychosis – a whole series of suppressed thoughts, which, thanks to the dream, more readily come to the scene of analysis.

# 3 Analogies between Dreams and Psychosis

This is perhaps the perspective from which the relationship between dreams and psychosis has been most extensively explored. As early as 1900/1971, Freud noted: "[...] attention was long ago directed to the underlying kinship between dreams and mental disorders, exhibited in the wide measure of agreement between their manifestations" (Freud, 1900/1971, pp.89–90).

In general terms, it could be said that the comparison between dreams and madness is long-standing. For Kant, the madman is a waking dreamer; for Schopenhauer, dreams are a brief madness and madness a long dream (cited by Freud, 1900/1971). Freud includes these comments, along with others of a similar nature, in his chapter on dreams and mental diseases, thereby opening a detailed review of the comparisons that classical psychiatry had drawn between these two phenomena up to that point. In his synthesis, we can find observations such as:

> Spitta (1882, 199), in much the same way as Maury (1854), enumerates as follows the different points of agreement which constitutes the basis for this comparison: '(1) Self-consciousness is suspended or at least retarded, which results in a lack of insight into the nature of the condition, with consequent inability to feel surprise and loss of moral consciousness. (2) Perception by the sense organs is modified: being diminished in dreams but as a rule greatly increased in insanity. (3) Interconnection of ideas occurs exclusively according to the laws of association and reproduction; ideas thus fall into sequences automatically and there is a consequent lack of proportion in the relation between ideas (exaggerations

DOI: 10.4324/9781003755166-5

> and illusions). All this leads to (4) an alteration or in some cases a reversal of personality and occasionally of character traits (perverse conduct).
>
> (Freud, 1900/1971, p.90)

The comparison continues with citations from other authors, which provide details such as the hallucinatory and coenesthetic quality of both phenomena, the salience of memories believed to be forgotten that emerge in both, and also the fulfilment of desire, which both dream representation and madness entail (Griesinger, cited by Freud, 1900/1971).

Radestock (cited in Freud, 1900/1971) points out that the rapid sequence of ideas in some dreams closely resembles the flight of ideas that afflicts some psychotic individuals; that the splitting of the dreamer's ego into various dream characters is similar to the personality splitting characteristic of certain psychoses; and that thought echo is akin to the voices anyone may hear during a dream. Likewise, he relates delusional fixed ideas to the stereotyped themes of recurring dreams.

Freud (1900/1971) concurs with all of this, going so far as to suggest that the study of dreams would be useful for revealing the internal mechanisms of mental diseases. This is, in fact, the common thread connecting his insights in *Die Traumdeutung* (1900/1971) with his study of Schreber's *Memoirs* (Freud, 1911/1981). In the former, Freud systematically addresses the mechanisms of displacement, condensation, and the means of dream representation, while in the latter, he focuses particularly on the role of condensation and distortion in the production of delusion.

Even many years later, Freud will continue to affirm that:

> the dream is a pathological product, the first member of the class which includes hysterical symptoms, obsessions and delusions, but [...] it is distinguished from the others by its transitoriness and by its occurrence under conditions which are part of normal life. [...]. The state of sleep involves a turning-away from the real external world, and there we have the necessary condition for the development of a psychosis. The most careful study of the severe psychoses will not reveal to us a single feature that is more characteristic of those pathological conditions.
>
> (Freud, 1933/1981, pp.15–16)

This comparison leads him to speak of the "harmless dream-psychosis" (p.16) and of the dream as a "harmless hallucinatory experience" (p.17).

In his seminar on psychoses (1955–56/1997) and in his doctoral thesis (1932), Lacan also introduces observations about the mechanisms and features akin to both dreams and psychosis. In his thesis, he goes considerably into the nature of delusional interpretation and, in several passages, compares it to dreams:

> Certain interpretations depend on physiological mechanisms akin to those of dreams. As is well known, in dreams the play of images seems to be set in motion, at least in part, by contact with the environment reduced to a minimum of pure sensation. Here, on the contrary, there is perception of the external world, but this perception presents a twofold alteration that assimilates it to the structure of dreams: it appears to us as tested in a psychical state intermediate between dreams and waking; furthermore, the threshold of belief, whose role is essential in perception, is here below its normal level.
> (Lacan, 1932, pp.125–126)

Beyond the common denominator of the belief the subject lends to the contents of their dreams – while asleep – and to their delusions, we see that Lacan points out the fact that both are built upon a minimal amount of information extracted from the environment, upon which the delusion or the dream scene is subsequently constructed.

A few pages later, continuing the inquiry into how dreams and delusions seek a way to integrate data from perception, he pauses to consider the phenomena of memory illusion and the creation of memory-images in psychosis – so similar to dream-work and, we might add, to the elaboration of screen memories in neurosis:

> If we wish to form a more precise picture of the mechanism of these illusions, let us think of a fact pertaining to dreams well known in psychology: the person suddenly awakened by a produced noise remembers having formed in dreams a concatenation of images whose culmination was that noise; they have the impression that the dream lasted a considerable time, and yet the entire *order of the concatenation is manifestly designed to incorporate the noise* – which was, in fact, what caused the awakening – and moreover the subject could not have foreseen either that the noise was coming

> or what form it would take. This fact, like all those that leave so enigmatic the problem of the duration of dreams, makes vividly apparent the difficulty that an objective temporal orientation presents in the representational unfolding of images.
>
> (p.128, italics added)

The paradoxical temporal arrangement that images receive, in both dreams and psychosis, is thus another coincidence that Lacan highlights, along with the tendentious nature of their concatenation – so apt at providing a symbolic framework for what comes from the real.

Another common point that he identifies between both phenomena is that delusion often allows us to observe the *inmixing of subjects*, just as in the dream of Irma's injection (Freud, 1900/1971). The practitioner colleagues whom Freud involves in that dream "are the between-I's", Lacan says, "who play an essential role here" (1955–56/1997, p.193); he then asks: "Isn't it precisely the inmixing of subjects that appears in delusion?" (p.194). To support the comparison, he invokes the characteristic confusion of wills that operates in delusion: "One *makes them do* this. This is where the problem lies [...]" (p.194; italics in original).

Lacan also compares the dream's navel to the delusional core of psychosis. In both cases, he argues, "the sense [...] appears to culminate in a hole" (p.260). In psychosis, it is meaning that is subtracted, yet at the same time presents itself as supremely full, in a flight that pulls the subject towards the core of the delusional phenomenon – its navel. In the dream, that navel situates the point at which nothing more can be extracted, "a knot, beyond which it is to the core of being that the dream appears to be attached" (p.260).

To conclude, let us say that these points of comparison – drawn by both classical psychiatry and psychoanalysis between dreams and psychosis – respond to a broader structure, more fully elaborated since Freud, in which psychical processes are shown to be products of certain laws of functioning, akin to all unconscious processes, and therefore, operative across every clinical structure.

# Part 2

# Dreams in Psychoses in Transference

The categorisation we have been following stems from Freud's attempt to classify a whole range of possible relations between dreams and *mental diseases* – let us recall that this was the term he used – and it has focused on the periods of crisis in psychoses.

We now turn to the clinical facts concerning dreams, though no longer as phenomena linked to the emergence, after-effects, or structure of the psychotic episode, but as trans-structural psychical acts of practical value for analytic treatments.

Until a few years ago, analytic literature rarely addressed the dreams brought to analysis by psychotic patients, their possible uses, or their relation to transference. "Do psychotics in transference also dream?", Daniel Paola asked in 1994, answering: "It is evident that they do, and moreover, that often a certain key lies therein" (p.66).

Everything we have said so far about the relationship between dreams and psychosis has been approached from a consideration of psychosis at its moments of destabilisation. Dreams therefore generally appeared in continuity or analogy with elementary phenomena – and indeed the two are closely intertwined during those periods – which is precisely what makes any questioning of the dream text more difficult.

A structural consideration of psychoses, however, compels us to also weigh the value of dreams during the extensive periods of life in which many psychotics neither hallucinate nor delude, or do so in a manner that does not prevent them from continuing an analytic treatment worthy of that name; as well as in the many cases of psychotics who never reach a point of destabilisation at all.

"Some psychotic subjects continue their analysis once the triggering has been overcome. The existence of dreams calls for an

DOI: 10.4324/9781003755166-6

intervention", asserted this author (Paola, 1994, p.70), a statement with which we concur.

In fact, when Freud reviewed the extensive medical literature on the relationship between dreams and mental disease, he concluded that research on one specific aspect of the topic remained largely unexplored: "Very little research has hitherto been carried out into the modifications occurring in dream-life during chronic psychoses" (1900/1971, p.89). At present, the advances made in this field – specifically in isolating dreams as an object of study – remain scarce.

As we mentioned earlier, in 1922/1981, Freud returned to this question in his paper on the mechanisms common to jealousy, paranoia, and homosexuality. In that text, he makes very interesting observations about the dreamer's relation to their dreams in two cases of paranoia. Having already examined the differential aspects of that text regarding how dream-life can be affected by psychosis, let us now pause on the more analytic aspects of the question. Freud writes:

> Dreams are distinguished from waking thought by the fact that they can include material (belonging to the region of the repressed) which must not emerge in waking thought. Apart from this, dreams are merely a *form of thinking*, a transformation of preconscious material of thought by the dream-work and its conditions. Our terminology of the neuroses is not applicable to repressed material; this cannot be called hysterical, nor obsessional, nor paranoic. As against this, the other part of the material which is subjected to the process of dream-formation – the preconscious thoughts – may be normal or may bear the character of any neurosis; they may be the products of any of the pathogenic processes in which the essence of a neurosis lies. There seems to be no reason why any such pathological idea should not be transformed into a dream. A dream may therefore quite simply represent a hysterical phantasy, an obsessional idea, or a delusion – that is, may reveal one or other of these upon interpretation.
>
> (pp.229–230)

We could say that in this paragraph, Freud not only distinguishes between what within the dream may be considered affected by the psychotic episode and what is not, but also offers an indication for analytic practice: interpretation could aim to reveal the obsessional, hysterical, or delusional idea upon which the dream was constructed.

That is to say, Freud – who at times discouraged the psychoanalysis of psychotic patients – nonetheless provides a guideline for it here, explaining that although "Cases of paranoia are for well-known reasons not usually amenable to analytic investigation [...] I have recently been able, nevertheless, by an intensive study of two paranoics, to discover something new to me" (p.225).

Let us now focus on another point in the cited paragraph: Freud highlights that dreams admit thoughts which, in waking life, would not emerge, and he demonstrates how this holds true for any clinical type. What does this tell us about psychotics in analysis? We believe it offers a valuable indication of the use we may make of the dreams that psychotic patients recount to us: within them lie thoughts that have not emerged openly in consciousness – or that have not yet emerged, as we saw in the section on dreams that introduce a psychotic episode – but which are there in potential, awaiting, so to speak, or in the making. Bringing them to light through the dream poses no greater danger than leaving them encysted; quite the contrary, for through their expression the analyst is enabled to intervene.

Freud, referring to his two paranoid patients, writes: "In both cases, therefore, the dream took up the material that was at the time *forced into the background* in waking life. This too, however, need not necessarily be an invariable rule" (p.230, italics added). We believe Freud's prudence here is inspired by what he himself had just pointed out regarding his limited experience with psychotic patients. But would we today refuse to elevate this to a rule? Is it not equally the case with psychotics that what has been *forced into the background* is what manifests in dreams?

# 4 What Unconscious? What Forms of Return?

## 4.1 That Which Has Been Forced Into The Background (*zurückgedrängt*)

It is worth pausing over the terminology Freud uses when speaking of the dreams of the paranoid patients he took into analysis. He says that the dream has gathered up, in both cases, what in waking life was at that moment being *forced into the background* (*zurückgedrängt*). This is not a term Freud employs frequently, although it appears in *Repression* (1915/2000a), to explain the action of repulsion, and in *The Interpretation of Dreams* (1900/1971), to describe the passage of a wish from the preconscious to the unconscious. Nevertheless, a more enigmatic use of this expression is found in *Totem and Taboo* (1913), where Freud explains that a mythological stage may be *surmounted* and *forced into the background* when another stage has come to replace it. It is thus linked to the problematic notion of that which has been *surmounted*, which Freud also employs in *The 'Uncanny'* (1919/1981), and which continues to raise questions for us regarding its distinction from the notion of the *repressed*.

It is not clear whether what is *forced into the background* should be equated with what is *repressed* (a notion to which Freud devoted a far greater degree of systematisation), since it appears to be an expression Freud employed only in rare occasions, and which, for some reason, he chose not to replace with *the repressed*.

In fact, a careful review of what Freud terms *the surmounted* in his text *The 'Uncanny'* offers a perspective on the complexity of situating or assigning a specific status to something that has not been exactly repressed and that, moreover, raises questions regarding the status that should be granted to it. For that which has been surmounted – does it

DOI: 10.4324/9781003755166-7

persist? Has it been preserved in some way? Does it hold a status of its own? Reading that text rather leads one to suppose that what has been surmounted remains in an indeterminate state, impossible to situate. The same problem arises with what has been *forced into the background* in *Totem and Taboo*: something has fallen out of reach, been lost, yet without Freud theorising any specific status for it.

Returning to the dreams of Freud's two paranoiac patients, we find that what was *forced into the background* was, in one case, the ideas preceding the episode – since that patient's dream "were quite normal while he was subject to his delusion" (Freud, 1922/1981, p.230) – and in the other, the delusional ideas, since his dream was "paranoic in content while he was treating his delusional ideas with contempt" (p.230). For this reason, Freud considers that in both cases the dreams gathered up what was *forced into the background*: that which, for the moment, forms no part of the analysand's discourse – what has not been admitted into consciousness.

This opens onto the broad and complex question of the differential mechanisms at play in the production of the unconscious in neurosis and psychosis.

In general terms, we know that in psychoanalysis repression (*Verdrängung*) – a mechanism that is in essence neurotic – is not regarded as coinciding with repudiation (*Verwerfung)*, which Freud formulated for the psychoses and which Lacan translated as *forclusion* (foreclosure in English). It therefore becomes necessary to determine whether what Freud calls *forced into the background* corresponds, in neurosis, to what we would regard as forming part of the repressed unconscious, or whether it should be instead considered as pertaining to what has been foreclosed.

In any case, what interests us here is not the status that might be attributed to that which has been *forced into the background* – which would lead us into metapsychology – but rather the rigorous determination of what mode of return is at play, for it is precisely there that clinical experiences reside. And not only the mode of return, but everything concerning the psychotic's position in relation to these returns – the stance they adopt in response to them.

As we shall see, the analysts who have most carefully examined the issue of dreams in psychoses advocate for a sustained distinction between what may return to the psychotic in the real – as loose signifiers, hallucinatory or delusional in nature – and what may reach them through the dream, which is always woven and, in some way, symbolised. What is at stake is a difference in the modes of return of that which has been rejected; and the whole question lies in how these returns are articulated in the encounter with an other – an analyst, for instance – where a discourse that is both sustained and heard can enable the inscription of something other than delusion and hallucination.

As we can see, we are now dealing with a more complex distinction than the one we initially took from Freud – that between the mechanisms of dream formation and the preconscious thoughts that serve as their material. We have entered a terrain where what comes into play is the dreamer's relation to their dream: their disposition to read it or to ignore it, to redirect it towards fruitful ground or to reject its content, to interpret it as a psychical act or as an external influence.

On this subject, we have published an article exploring Freudian observations and findings from the pass regarding the relationship of neurotic dreamers with their dreams at different moments of treatment (Labaronnie & Lombardi, 2018). There, we distinguished three positions: a defensive one, a more open one, and a decided position characteristic of advanced analyses.

We now find that these observations on the neurotic analysand's relationship with their dreams are by no means remote from what occurs with psychotic analysands. As we shall see, the cases reported by several analysts support this line of thought, in which it becomes possible to distinguish different moments in the appropriation – or, more precisely, the reading – of dream material, even in psychoses.

## 4.2 The Excluded, the Ignored, the Unassumed

It's classically said that in psychosis the unconscious is at the surface, conscious. This is even why articulating it doesn't seem to have much effect. [...] Its being articulated doesn't imply its *recognition*, though. [...] If it's ever possible for someone to speak in a language that he is totally *ignorant* of, we can say that the psychotic subject is ignorant of the language he speaks.

Is this a satisfactory metaphor? Certainly not. The question is not so much why this unconscious, which is articulated at ground level, remains *excluded* for the subject, *not adopted* by him – but why it appears in the real (Lacan, 1955-56/1997, pp.11–12, our italics).

With this assertion, Lacan produces a change of direction: he does not set out to investigate "why this unconscious, which is articulated at ground level, remains *excluded* for the subject, *not adopted* by him", since his interest at that time was focused on explaining why the unconscious appears for the psychotic in the real. We must now take the reverse path, for our question is precisely this: why does that which is articulated *out in the open* (Lacan, 1955-56/1997, p.59) remain excluded for the psychotic subject?

We would say that what is at stake here is the psychotic's position-taking. We believe this is the correct way to understand the famous rejection of the unconscious by the psychotic (Lacan, 1973). We shall also see that a number of contemporary analysts maintain that such rejection can change over the course of an analysis (see Section 5.2). But why would a psychotic subject wish to reconsider the position they have taken with respect to what we may call, in general terms, "the rejected"? Freud offers us an approach in the following observation:

> In paranoia, self-reproach is repressed in a manner which may be described as *projection.* It is repressed by erecting the defensive symptom of *distrust of other people.* In this way the subject withdraws his acknowledgement of the self-reproach; and, as if to make up for this, he is deprived of a protection against the self-reproaches which return in his delusional ideas.
>
> (Freud, 1896/1999, p.184, italics in original)

Freud thus introduces the idea that projection effectively serves to ignore and exclude a thought-content, while clarifying that such exclusion will not occur without returns. What has been ignored will return by way of delusion or hallucination, taking the form of insult, persecution, or indignity – in short, the obscene and ferocious face of the superego.

> The problem is that evidently the unconscious, rejected in neurosis, in common discourse, or in psychosis, continues to affect. What does 'to affect' mean here, and what is affected? Whom does it affect? The one affected here is not the subject; what is affected is the body, it is the body's jouissance.
>
> (Soler, 2004, p.245)

For this reason, when Freud (1894/1981a, p.58) pointed out that repudiation or rejection constitutes "a much more energetic and successful kind of defence" than repression, he also warned of its high cost, since "from the moment at which this has been successfully done the subject is in a psychosis, which can only be classified as 'hallucinatory confusion'" (p.58). The success in question lies in dismissing a thought with the same radicality as the affect accompanying it; yet everything suggests that both – thought and affect – are subsequently encountered again through other channels: in the suffering brought about by hallucinatory persecution, or in the surplus suffering of the paranoiac, who rediscovers everywhere, projected onto others, what they have denied.

The situation is quite different, in our view, when what returns to the psychotic comes by way of the dream. Reproach will not be absent there either, but one could say it can attain a logical form closely resembling the neurotic's subjective rectification – a kind of response to the question: *What is your own involvement in the mess you complain of?* (see Sections 9.6.2 and 9.6.7).

There is an elaboration in what returns by way of the dream, unlike in the hallucinatory return. It is therefore very different for the psychotic to receive the hallucinatory accusation "Sow!" (Lacan, 1955-56/1997, p.62) than to receive in a dream the statement "you're the one who starts all the arguments" (see Section 9.6.2). The former is an injurious utterance that objectifies; the latter leaves some space for a subject who may wish to recognise that therein lies a certain key for modifying their situation within the social bond.

As regards the psychotic's initial position-taking, however, we can recognise a coincidence in both cases: they will say, "that's not mine"; that is, it concerns them, but it is not theirs – it is something sent from the outside.

# 5 On the Rejection of the Unconscious in the Psychoses

## 5.1 A Very Special Inertia

"Our starting point is this – the unconscious is present but not functioning. Contrary to what has been thought, the fact that it's present doesn't imply a solution but, on the contrary, *a very special inertia*" (Lacan, 1955–56/1997, pp.143–144, italics added).

The unconscious is present, but not functioning. Its presence does not make it any less unreadable for the psychotic. Perhaps it is precisely because it is present – so out in the open – that the psychotic rejects it, preferring not to read it. Or, conversely, perhaps it is because the psychotic takes up a position of rejection, that it returns to them again and again, at times in a raw and unmediated way. The point is that this paints a picture in which it is very often the other who reads something in what returns to the psychotic – it is the other of the social bond who finds obvious the relation between the psychotic and what besieges them.

> In short, it could be said that the psychotic is a martyr of the unconscious, giving this term *martyr* its meaning, which is to be a witness. It's an open testimony. The neurotic is also a witness to the existence of the unconscious, he gives a closed testimony that has to be deciphered. The psychotic, in the sense in which he is in a first approximation an open witness, seems arrested, immobilized, in a position that leaves him incapable of authentically restoring the sense of what he witnesses and sharing it in the discourse of others.
> (Lacan, 1955–56/1997, p.132)

If we set aside for a moment the fact that what is at stake here is a return in the real, we can discern that the clinical problem posed by

DOI: 10.4324/9781003755166-8

such a return is, ultimately, what to do with that which cannot and does not wish to be read. From this angle, these reflections on what appears in an open testimony – yet is not therefore legible, and, above all, not shareable within discourse – come very close to the problem. Lacan (1962–63) formulated a few years later as that of *acting out*. There is truth there, but it is not interpretable – at least not at first – either by the analyst or by the subject. The problem then becomes, as Lacan puts it, "how the horse is to be made to walk the lunge ring, to trot round the pen" (p.126); that is, how to set in motion, along readable and transferential paths, that which at the outset is truth without a subject.

Allowing for the differences, we believe that this is the same problem Lacan encounters in his conceptualisation of the fantasy (*fantasme*): the subject, like the hero of Greek tragedy, enacts a script they do not know – one that is evident to those around him, there in plain sight, but which has been unable to be read. The entire analysis will be devoted to delineating and bringing to light the text of which it is composed, until it reaches a point of writing – that of the axiom of the fantasy – which, for the first time, makes possible a reading of the structure underlying the drama.

We will see, in the case of C., that the first dream to arise in analysis presents a kind of wild subjective rectification, for she receives from her own dream the message that it is she – and not her jouissant Other – who starts the arguments. This dream surprises the analyst by its transparency. Yet as soon as it is questioned, it receives from the dreamer a radical disavowal: that dream contains no truth whatsoever; it is merely an accusation.

It will be through subjective destitution that the analyst will be able to make a detour, awaiting the moment when the truth the psychotic has yet to find can emerge – when they are able to hear it.

## 5.2 Reconciliation, Hystericisation, Saying, and Transindividuality

For several years now, a number of analysts have ventured to question the status of the unconscious in psychoses (Apollon, 2008a, 2008b; Bergeron, 2008; Boukhabza, 2012, 2013; Cantin, 2008; De Battista, 2015; Lombardi & Laje, 2016; Vetere, 2014). It has begun to be considered that, through the encounter with an analyst, the psychotic individual can review and modify their position towards the unconscious. Julieta de Battista explains that "this would not alter the initial choice, the forced choice, but it would allow us to consider a modalisation of the rejection or a modification of the position through the encounter with the function of the analyst's desire" (p.218). In this way, she raises the question of the psychotic's relationship with the unconscious, as mediated by the transferential encounter:

> The question is whether the invitation offered by psychoanalysis might provide an opportunity for the psychotic to reposition themselves in relation to the structure and make progress in understanding their symptom – that is, in the know-how in relation to it. To exchange the initial flight from the unconscious for a reconciliation.
> (p.222)

In this same vein, Gabriel Lombardi (2018) has been advocating for the necessity of passing through the hysterical discourse to make analysis possible across every clinical type: neurosis, psychosis, or perversion. The analytic discourse thus becomes a generator of hystericisation in the analysand, provided that the analyst has been able to destitute themselves as a subject and adopt a submissive stance towards the subjective position of the one consulting them.

> On condition of destituting himself as a subject to the point of achieving a 'strict submission to all the subjective positions' of the paranoiac, the analyst can receive him, gain his trust – even his complicity – so that he may open his unconscious to him and become divided, and weep in session, and eventually pass from dreams of persecution to dreams of dissatisfaction. And resume his life, his work, and certain bonds of friendship and love, in his own way.
> (Lombardi, 2018, p.80)

All the works that suggest this possibility of hystericisation and of working with the unconscious in psychoses emphasise the enabling function of the encounter with an analyst. We may also cite other variants that situate the issue on the basis of other elements of Lacan's teaching.

> How can a new subject be brought into being where the 'unsoundable decision of being' (Lacan, 1946/1985) structures him as the subject of an obligatory freedom? Far from being the final word, the so-called 'foreclosure of the Name-of-the-Father'

> provides an indication of how enunciation is structured, but says nothing, precisely, about the scope of the saying of a speaking being following the encounter with an analyst.
>
> (Lombardi and Laje, 2016, p.113)

What we have here is a questioning of the position adopted towards the unconscious in psychoses that proceeds from the notions of *enunciation* and *saying*, precisely in order to indicate that transference might influence the scope of that saying.

We also find a similar proposal in Vetere (2014), which, starting from the postulate of the transindividuality of the unconscious, suggests that in the encounter with an analyst the unconscious as "discourse of the Other" may shift from the objective genitive – we are spoken by the Other, by its discourse; a truth laid bare in psychotic crises – to the subjective genitive – the unconscious as a discourse that speaks about the Other, situating and circumscribing its marks, the signifiers it has offered. "The analysis of a subject can only be brought about with an analyst. This is a reminder to us that the unconscious is essentially speech, speech of the other, and can only be recognized when the other sends it back to you" (Lacan, 1955–56/1997, p.241).

This postulate of the transindividuality of the unconscious also makes it possible to conceive of work with psychotic patients as giving rise to an unconscious of ethical status – an unconscious situated in what is said and in how that saying is heard within the framework of a certain bond.

> This transindividuality of the unconscious -likely suggested to Lacan through his entry into psychoanalysis by way of psychosis – is [...] sustained throughout his entire body of work. He thus invites us to locate the unconscious nowhere other than in what we say, and since all speech is framed within a relation of interlocution, the unconscious is not inside anyone but resides on the surface of the discourse that unfolds between the subject and the Other. In this way, a novel conception of the unconscious is formulated, one which fundamentally questions Freud's endopsychic model.
>
> (Vetere, 2014, pp.169–170)

The perspectives detailed above by no means exhaust current proposals, but they serve as a small sample of a body of work that, drawing on different theoretical resources, points towards a possible modalisation of the psychotic's initial rejection of the unconscious.

### 5.3 Reading and Writing

On 10 January 1978, Lacan reflected in his seminar in the following terms:

> There is surely writing in the unconscious, if only because the dream, the principle of the unconscious – that's what Freud said – the lapses and even the witticism are defined by the readable. One has a dream, one does not know why, and then subsequently it is read; the same with a slip, and everything that Freud says about witticism is quite notorious as being linked to this economy which is writing, economy as compared to speech. The readable – that is what knowledge consists of. And in short, it is limited. What I say about the transference is that I timidly advanced it as being the subject – a subject always supposed, there is no subject, of course, there is only the supposed – the supposed-to-know. What could that mean? The *supposed-to-know-how-to-read-otherwise* (*autrement*).
>
> (Lacan, 1977–78, 10 January 1978, pp.24–25)

The proposal for transference that may be deduced from this is, therefore, to *know how to read otherwise* (Vetere, 2014, p.172).

Why does it become necessary to situate analytic practice at the level of a *know-how-to-read*? We believe it is because Lacan insisted, from the outset, on the superficiality of the unconscious, on its participation in all discourse, on its character as "[...] not so much deep as it is inaccessible to conscious scrutiny [...]" (Lacan, 1957, p.364). If the unconscious is within reach – if it is, like the purloined letter, in full view of all – why would anyone undertake an analysis? The answer, we believe, lies in this indication given by Lacan: in order to learn to read, and above all to read otherwise what, subjected to a repetitive, delusional, or alienating reading, produces a surplus of suffering that may be circumscribed.

This perhaps makes it possible to understand why, even though psychosis evidently presents an "unconscious out in the open" – that of delusion and hallucination – we nonetheless continue to encounter psychotics who wish to recount their dreams and who find, in the analyst's response, a new reading with pacifying and vitalising effects. This virtue of analysis with psychotic patients, of course, is not limited to work with dreams; yet it allows us to resolve the paradox whereby what presents itself out in the open nonetheless often needs to be read – and, for that, it must return by other pathways.

That which is *forced into the background*, which Freud discerned in the dreams of his two paranoiac patients, if recounted in transference, can be intervened upon.

Moreover, the interpretative character of the dream itself does not prevent it from being interpreted – or *read*, one might say – in a second turn. As Lacan indicates: "retroactively, that is read".

The writing carried out by the work of the unconscious, as well as its reading, produce effects upon *jouissance* – a question to which we shall return.

# 6 Contributions to a Possible Work with Dreams in Psychoses

In addition to the proposals that have been gaining ground concerning the status of the unconscious in psychoses and the possible modalisations of its rejection – possible reconciliations, hystericisation, the putting-into-discourse, the possibility of a saying – there are also several works by analysts that have begun to draw attention to the importance dreams may acquire in analytic treatments with psychotic patients. Dominique Boukhabza, former Head of the Mental Health Service at the Valvert Hospital in Marseille, comments:

> For several years now, numerous works have made advances concerning the treatment of psychotic patients and, in each case, within those advances the dream played a primordial role; it was a lever in the progress of the treatment. [...] In what way does the dream constitute such a lever? That is what we shall attempt to develop.
>
> (2013, p.185)

The works she mentions (Apollon, 2008a, 2008b; Bergeron, 2008; Cantin, 2008; Kolko, 2004) have been devoted both to theorising the role of the dream and to reporting certain analytic treatments presenting uses of dreams which, only a few decades ago, would have been contraindicated.

Although at one time the psychotic dream was equated with delusion, these authors now propose to separate these strands, distinguishing the place the dream affords the subject from the place offered by delusion. A similar question arises with regard to hallucinations: are the voices that present themselves as a return in the real equivalent to those the

DOI: 10.4324/9781003755166-9

psychotic may report as having formed part of a dream? We shall say that they are not. Indeed, the clinical and theoretical demonstrations offered by these authors make it possible to draw lines of separation aimed at avoiding any confusion between the return in the real and dream elaboration – the latter, on the contrary, having proved to be an effective remedy against the former. According to Boukhabza, the displacement of elements of delusion or hallucination into the scene of the dream – that Other scene constitutive of the unconscious – enables the subject to recognise them as their own and to work through them in a different manner. At this point, the heteronomous origin that Schreber attributed to all his dreams is instructive of a subjective position that would not be compatible with dream analysis – though this does not imply that such a position cannot change following the establishment of transference, which grants the unconscious a different discursive place.

## 6.1 Dreams in the Establishment of Transference and the Inauguration of a Position of Not-Knowing

As these authors demonstrate, dreams – even in cases of psychosis – can bear witness to the establishment of transference and to the analysand's formulation of a demand for analysis arising from the encounter with an analyst. Such is the case of the "dream of the voices", reported by Boukhabza in the treatment of a patient referred to as A.: "I have bugs in my ears; I remove them. When there are no more left, I wake up" (2013, p.186). The dreamer points out that after removing the bugs he was able to hear properly. The analyst takes up the question of hearing; the analysand then states: "The voices, I would like them to stop" (p.186). In her book, the analyst draws attention to the fact that the awakening does not occur because of the voices, but because of their absence. "The dream of the voices indicates a direction: that of the elaboration of a knowledge in the place of, and as a substitute for, the voices. This knowledge is produced by the dream-work" (p.186).

As the author notes, the establishment of transference implies, first and foremost, a position on the part of the analyst that presupposes a knowledge in the psychotic subject – a knowledge to be learned from him. Only subjective destitution on the side of the analyst can enable this possibility.

Yet the question of knowledge cannot remain at that point, for it is precisely through the establishment of transference that the reopening of the hole in language – the incompleteness of the Other – becomes possible; a hole that delusion had attempted to plug. In the dream of the voices, the term used to name the bugs, *bêtes*, resonates with *bêta* (fool, stupid), "the one who does not know" (p.186), as the author points out. Transference thereby allows for a certain distance from the certainty of meaning that afflicts the psychotic. Moreover, that Other of the psychotic, who knows everything, may also be rendered incomplete, for in analysis both analysand and analyst must allow themselves to be taught by the unconscious.

In this way, the work of delusion is progressively replaced by analytic work, in which the unconscious participates in a different manner:

> In order to displace the axis of psychotic work, to redirect it towards an interest in the dream, in order to create an enthusiasm for the discoveries that the work of the dream will bring, we first listen attentively to the psychotic analysand as they explain the particularities of their experience; we identify the events that have placed the work of delusion in jeopardy and provoked the crisis, and we take the delusional experience as seriously as, for example, the verbalisation of suicidal ideas. We must be well acquainted with the analysand's reason for living, what defines the meaning of their life – sometimes from early childhood – before encouraging the work of deconstructing the delusional system through the fragments of history that dreams will contribute. The analyst will thus allow the analysand's own dream to 'comment on' and interrogate the delusion, to introduce doubts into it, to call the voices into question. Progressively, the dream comes to diminish the delusion and, little by little, a subjective history takes shape, with the aim of becoming the new point of support for life.
>
> (Bergeron, 2008, p.243)

What emerges from this is a necessary passage from certainty of meaning – as a position with regard to knowledge – to a *not-knowing* that inaugurates analysis. Within this perspective we may also situate the transition from the persecutory dreams of the paranoiac to dreams of dissatisfaction – a transformation which, as we mentioned in Section 5.2, has been pointed out by Lombardi (2018). One of the cases reported by Cantin includes a dream of this kind, in which the effect of the hystericisation of a paranoiac – an effect that renders him analysable – can be observed:

> I must repair a bicycle for my neighbour. It is a white bicycle. She tells me she has no money, but that I can pay for the parts myself and that she will reimburse me. But I realise that the shop is closed and that I will not be able to do it.
>
> (Cantin, 2008, p.190)

A dream strikingly similar to that of the Butcher's Wife (Freud, 1900/1971, p.147), it coincides in staging what is impeded, unsatisfied, unfinished. The analyst comments that it provided the opportunity to speak about certain moments in this analysand's life in which personal projects had been cut short. The abandonment of those projects had entailed the adoption of a position after which the elementary phenomena had intensified. This brings us to the question of historisation in the analysis of psychotics and to the way in which dreams may contribute to this task.

## 6.2 Dreams and Historisation

Another point of interest in the works we have been discussing concerns historisation. With each dream, new files of memories are opened and set into dialogue. The elements of the dream refer back to scenes from the subject's history, enabling these to enter into the transference, to be commented upon and ordered – a work we shall not hesitate to regard as one of writing.

In his thesis, Lacan offered the following example:

> All the characteristic features of Aimée's behaviour are brought together in this account: she delayed over her personal preparations while the others, having completed the arrangements for a joint outing, had already left the house; in order to catch up with them, she took a path across open country and had the clumsiness to provoke a bull, from which she escaped by a hair's breadth. This theme of the bull charging to attack reappears frequently in Aimée's dreams (alongside a dream of a viper, an animal that abounds in her native land), and it is always of ill omen. The theme likewise appears in her writings. Perhaps a psychoanalyst might succeed in penetrating further into the determinism of that event, into its

> affective and imaginative sequelae, and might discover subtle symbolic relations between those elements.
>
> (Lacan, 1932, p.134)

Yet it is not only the recollections of ordinary experiences that may be explored through their presentation in dreams; experiences of estrangement will likewise often be taken up again by the work of the dream. "The dream will allow the exploration of the decisive moments in the subject's life in which they were confronted with some defect in the structure of reality", says Apollon (2008b, p.39).

The dream thereby takes up the elements of delusion by a route closer to historisation, making it possible to grasp the subjective truth – the real kernel that delusion had enveloped in its imaginary covering. Apollon (2008a, 2008b) maintains that the dream will take up hallucinatory experiences and their linkage with certain memories, an idea with which we concur. Cantin (2008) likewise affirms that dreams make it possible, in the analysis of psychotic patients, to arrive at constructions that reorganise in a new way the earliest memories and psychical events, the psychotic experiences dating from childhood or adolescence, the thoughts that traversed psychotic moments, and the acts staged during crises. "It is the dream and its associations that will have brought the psychotic individual back to the moment when that thought first arose, to the context in which it appeared or imposed itself" (Cantin, 2008, p.189).

In addition to the cases we shall examine in the clinical sections, we find a related example in the case history of the Wolf Man. There, Freud finds that the famous dream of the wolves seated in a walnut-tree, seen through a window, takes up certain hallucinatory experiences through the element of the *walnut-tree*. The patient recalls:

> When I was five years old, I was playing in the garden near my nurse, and *was carving with my pocket-knife in the bark of one of the walnut-trees that come into my dream as well*. Suddenly, to my unspeakable terror, I noticed that I had cut through the little finger of my (right or left?) hand, so that it was only hanging on by its skin. I felt no pain, but great fear. I did not venture to say anything to my nurse, who was only a few paces distant, but I sank down on the nearest seat and sat there incapable of casting another glance at my finger. At last I calmed down, took a look at the finger, and saw that it was entirely uninjured.
>
> (Freud, 1918, p.85, italics added)

This memory of a hallucination, experienced with immense anguish at a very early age, is connected to the dream through the inclusion of the walnut-tree. A second hallucinatory experience is later recalled, likewise through its connection with a tree:

> In telling the story again on a later occasion he made the following correction: 'I don't believe I was cutting the tree. That was a confusion with another recollection, which must also have been hallucinatorily falsified, of having made a cut in a tree with my knife and of *blood* having come out of the tree'.
>
> (Freud, 1918, p.85, fn.2)

Although the Wolf Man's diagnosis is a matter that has given rise to much debate (Escars, 2002), and one we do not intend to settle here, it is worthwhile pausing over this connection between the famous dream and the two hallucinatory experiences that may have emerged from its interrogation – especially since the analysts who have published work on dreams in psychoses emphasise precisely how frequently dreams take up the earliest hallucinatory experiences, the first dramatic junctures, and experiences of estrangement.

These analysts regard the dream as a privileged means of transmission, insofar as it enables the psychotic to move towards increasingly communicable formulations of the experience of the irruption of the real. Through the associations arising from its fragments, the dream also collaborates in the construction of a history compatible with the social bond. It brings forth the recollection of events, signifiers of the symbolic Other that have marked the life of that subject, knowledge both constructed and yet to be constructed, which will no longer remain isolated and detached, and which, by virtue of this transformation, will cease to return as voices or delusional certainties.

> In short, the dream, as an unconscious act, will have means at its disposal of which conscious language is deprived. Thus, from the moment of their arrival at the Centre [*Centre psychanalytique de traitement pour adultes psychotiques* «388»], the psychotic knows what a psychoanalysis will entail and that, for this, he will have to make of his dreams a means of work.
>
> (Apollon, 2008a, p.69, our brackets)

The value of dreams in these treatments is manifold: while they make it possible to work through the traumatic real, they also introduce the possibility of speaking about certain memories or current circumstances, functioning as a vector of speech.

## 6.3 Three Moments in the Psychotic's Relationship with Their Dreams

While some analysts consider that the psychotic's difficulty in associating to be an obstacle to working with dream material (Capozzi & De Masi, 2001), Apollon (2008a, 2008b), Bergeron (2008) and Cantin (2008) advocate distinguishing three moments in the relation that the psychotic analysand will have to their dreams.

The first corresponds to the already mentioned lack of differentiation between dream and delusion, or dream and hallucination – the situation most frequently reported in the literature discussed in the first part of this work.

According to these authors, at this stage the psychotic is not yet concerned by their own speech. The position of rejection of the unconscious is maintained. Delusional certainty blocks and prevents the opening of a not-knowing in relation to the unconscious, and the dream therefore emerges undifferentiated and without palpable consequences.

Mr. R., treated by Lucie Cantin, illustrates this well. Asked to recount his dreams in analysis, he brings material that is nothing other than a continuation of the delusion: "there is a new weapon for the UN, they are small pellets with cannons from which they are fired; that was flying through the air like satellites that remain in orbit; that was attacking a rebel army" (Cantin, 2008, p.188). He then explains that he himself is a mediator in that entire conflict between countries, the UN, and the rebel armies. "The psychotic presents what he calls a dream, but which is in fact nothing more than the continuation of the interpretation produced by the imaginary of the delusion that he continues to elaborate", the author comments (p.188).

Another of her analysands states the following: "I doubt everything; my name is the only thing I do not doubt. The dreams I have … I have the impression that they are memories and not dreams" (p.194). When the analyst asks why he has that impression, the patient explains:

> because within me I have a feeling of déjà vu and déjà vécu (already seen and already lived). Every day I have that feeling. It piles up

> with myths, rumours, the films I have seen, with my experiences, my memories, the people I have known.
>
> (p.194)

Here we encounter once again the much-discussed continuity between dream and waking life in psychosis, only that in this example this state of affairs is explained with remarkable clarity by this analysand, who is not entirely overtaken by the confusion but is able to speak about it directly, perhaps even to symptomatise it.

The second moment already involves a certain entry of the dream into the transferential bond. Its contents are no longer confused with those of hallucination or delusion, yet neither do they carry, for the psychotic, legible consequences. It is rather a matter of the unfolding of an unconscious logic that the psychotic is learning to sustain by a route distinct from that of delusion, but which does not yet suffice for interpretation – on the part of the dreamer – nor is it reached by it when it comes from the analyst.

> I could specify this moment of the treatment, when the dream does no more than sustain the subject's speech within the experience, by saying that the chains, the connections, are formed in the analyst and not on the side of the psychotic. It is in the analyst, in effect, that the first elements of a logic are gradually located.
>
> (Cantin, 2008, p.191)

This moment strikes us as particularly significant, for it is possible to recognise in it the shaping of the unconscious within the transferential bond, without there being any passage through consciousness of what the dream might contribute – a question to which we shall return.

In accounting for the existence of a third moment in the psychotic analysand's relation to their dreams, these authors concur that although the first dreams to emerge in treatment will merely continue the delusional elaboration, at some point a dream will appear that responds to the analyst's desire – to their questions, to their position of allowing themselves to be taught by the psychotic – and that will serve to organise certain memories and associations according to a logic different from that of delusion. A "true dream", says Cantin, "which is no longer assimilable to the delusional elaboration" (p.192).

> What does the dream teach you about yourself? What does it make you recall from your past, from what you have lived through?' the

> analyst might ask, or even 'What does your unconscious convey to you through this dream about the difficulties you have encountered in the past? What disturbing impression or unbearable experience might have produced this nightmare?
>
> (Bergeron, 2008, pp.243–244)

We thus have a first moment, marked by a certain continuity and lack of differentiation between dream and delusion; a second, in which it is the analyst who apprehends the new logic that the dreams introduce; and a third, in which the psychotic is at last able to hear that new logic, to appropriate their oneiric production, to question it and to associate.

> In response to the analyst's desire to know, the dream's signifiers can reveal a subjective position previously concealed by the delusional organisation. [...] The dream's signifiers, directed towards the analyst –who refrains from making any demands and interpretations– are discovered and recognised with surprise by the analysand as part of their own Unconscious. These signifiers are going to progressively call into question the delusion that sustained the subject's submission to the jouissance of the Other.
>
> (Bergeron, 2008, p.232)

According to these authors, at this point some patients decide to interrupt the treatment. Others, on the contrary, reaffirm their commitment to the analysis and benefit from its effects. Those who abandon it often state clearly that they do not wish to lose the certainty they possessed (in their delusion) – those truths experienced as their sole support in life. Those who choose to continue consent to inaugurate a position of not-knowing, one that is genuinely unprecedented for the psychotic. Many confess that it is precisely because their ideas have been shaken in analysis that they find it necessary to continue. "Analytic work will replace the work of psychosis", comments Apollon (2008a, p.70). The dream gives rise to the production of a new knowledge – a "creative word" (Cantin, 2008, p.187) – emerging from the encounter with the analyst's not-knowing. This analytic work, oriented towards the possibility of apprehending one's own subjective position, provides the psychotic with other tools of reading than those of delusion.

As in neurosis, analysis must illuminate, bring to light, elucidate the subject's elective position, thereby promoting shifts in position capable of modifying the mortifying side of repetition. In this way, progress may also be made towards the possibility of naming that edge between the symbolic and the real which might circumscribe the delusional or hallucinatory experience. It is in this direction that dreams will make their greatest contributions.

> The dream triumphs where delusion runs aground. [...] The dream 'triumphs' when it succeeds in producing a symbolisation, a representation that evokes in the signifier what was at stake in that ill encounter with the real. It is not, therefore, just any dream that triumphs. [Only that which succeeds in] treating the real.
>
> (p.187, our brackets)

For our part, we consider it important to maintain, in relation to the difference between the second and third moments, a line of questioning concerning the role of consciousness in psychoanalytic treatments, both of neurotics and of psychotics. We advocate the hypothesis that effects in analysands are already very noticeable from the first moment transference is properly established, and that it is not necessary to wait for *insight* or a passage through consciousness to observe that libidinal effects, at the level of the symptom and of the act, manifest through the work with the unconscious itself. We believe that in the analysis of psychotics this is even more striking, for the rejection of the unconscious appears to originate and be maintained at the level of consciousness, while at the unconscious level something has already been set to work – something that the analyst hears and whose effects they observe. We consider this observable in the texts of Bergeron (2008) and Cantin (2008), whose clinical accounts allow one to appreciate that even in advanced treatments the associations the psychotic may make on the basis of their dreams are not always evident, whereas the effects they derive from them – whether or not they are aware of this – clearly are. We will return to this thesis in connection with case C. (Chapter 9).

Boukhabza (2012) does not emphasise as much as the Canadian authors the distinction between a second and a third moment – that is, a supposed passage between a period in which only the analyst apprehends the connections and the subjective truth revealed by the psychotic's dreams, and a third in which the patient would have acquired a certain ability to associate and to read their dreams. She emphasises instead that associations must be sought in subsequent dreams, a point to which we will return in the following section.

In our view, some psychotics show themselves, from the outset, very capable of reading in their dreams thoughts that can be connected with waking life – both present and past – while others go through long stretches of analysis without acquiring this ability, despite showing great interest in their dreams and being very productive dreamers. It will not escape anyone that, in this respect, the same occurs from one neurotic to another. Yet perhaps in psychosis this rupture between the unconscious and consciousness must be taken even more seriously. As we have said, the key to a successful analysis cannot rest upon *insight* or conscious reflections; rather, we recognise its progress through the libidinal effects that are either reported by the patient or observed by ourselves within the transference.

To illustrate two markedly different positions in relation to the reading of one's own dreams, I will briefly mention two situations involving psychotic patients whose analysis I conducted.

Mrs. D., aged 56, seeks consultation after a lifetime of psychiatric treatments for her manic-depressive episodes. Her melancholic side is striking, filled with self-reproaches about a wide variety of matters, together with a loss of the sense of vitality since her father's death some years ago, and the reports from her therapeutic companions, who mention that she does not bathe, cook, tidy, or clean her home.

Once she begins to feel at ease, she mentions an erotomaniac delusion binding her to her psychiatrist, and confesses not knowing "how she ought to conduct herself" in relation to him.

After some time in treatment with me, I ask her whether she dreams. She says that she has been dreaming a great deal lately, always about her parents, but cannot remember anything in particular. "What a pity", I say, "not even a single detail?" – to which she replies, very amiably, that yes, she does remember one. "My mum was there, and she gave me a little baby, very tiny" (she gestures with her hands, forming a bowl-like shape, indicating a diminutive size). Then she adds: "well, it wasn't a fully formed baby; it was like what comes before the baby forms. And she gave it to me". She searches for the word, cannot find it, and eventually settles on embryo or fetus. I ask her what she thinks about this dream, to which she replies, quite candidly: "That baby must be me; I need to start over from scratch". She is referring to something we had been discussing: following her father's death she has struggled to find motivation, projects, or ways to manage. That loss devastated her life; grief and self-reproach consumed her. By the time she recounts the dream, however, I point out several things she has recently been doing that used to be far more difficult. She replies: "The danger of death is over now; that's done, that's behind me. Now I need to figure out what I want to do".

I believe that she leaves that session with a guiding idea, given by her own dream. And I come away with the discovery that D. naturally assumes a readable connection between her dreams and her life.

The case of E. is different: a committed dreamer, aged twelve, brought for consultation because of "episodes of psychomotor agitation" – the psychiatrist's words – at school and at home. During one of these crises he shouted, "who said that adults are the ones who make the rules!" – and remembers nothing of it. He accepts that the adults have told me the truth about these episodes, but cannot recall them himself beyond a few details. He shows no interest in speaking about almost anything, until I discover that he is interested in his dreams. In everything else he is extremely terse, finding it difficult to construct sentences and often preferring an indifferent "I don't know".

Shortly after he begins to recount his dreams, a demand for analysis emerges which I read on the basis of one of them: there are people mixed together, faces that melt, people joined to their ghosts – which are like shadows – and the mission in the dream is to separate them. He dreams almost every week and remembers many details; he even creates a blog, with a friend's help, to recount one of his dreams. He tells me that years ago he began to hear the occasional voice and that at times he sees things "that aren't there". His hallucinations are taken up again in his dreams, inserted into new plots that allow an orientation to be read.

What stands out in E. is his interest in the dream narrative and its details. He associates a previous dream with a new one and attends to recurring elements, yet is completely incapable of associating anything from his dreams with his waking life – such connections arise only if I suggest them. Despite fairly guided questions, his aptitude for the oneiric contrasts sharply with his difficulty to reflect on his everyday life. Unlike what we will see with C., however, the connections I suggest to E. are almost always well received by him and reaffirmed once I articulate them. His position is not one of rejection of interpretation but of an incapacity to produce it himself. Perhaps this notable difference between C. and E. has to do with the fact that in the latter we are dealing with schizophrenia, whereas C., as we shall see, displays a decidedly paranoid structure.

This brief mention of two dissimilar cases – E. and Mrs. D. – has served to illustrate two very different positions in relation to dreams, even though both display notable abilities for working with dream material. In E., one can appreciate more clearly the rupture between an unconscious that works admirably and a consciousness that tends to remain unaware of that entire process.

We thus contrast the postulation of three moments in the psychotic's relation to their dreams with the proposal that what is at stake is rather different positions and different inclinations among psychotics, who are always very different from one another. Nevertheless, we believe that the postulation of three moments makes it possible to appreciate clinical subtleties which, in some patients, truly mark differential phases – moments of opening towards possibilities of working with their dreams that had previously been entirely absent.

As a final example, let us return to our dear Schreber. The belief that his dreams come from the divine rays coexists, in his case, with a notable ability to read them – as can be appreciated if we return to one of his footnotes, cited previously, where he recounts a dream and alerts us to how we should understand some of its oneiric elements:

> From the content of these notes I will here only quote that according to the vision produced by miracle in my dream, an attendant of the Asylum, whom I had first heard opening the door of the living-room adjoining my bedroom, was partly sitting on my bed, partly getting up to some mischief near my bed, at one time *eating smoked tongue or ham with beans*; that I saw myself still in the dream vision having left the bed in order to turn on the light so that the miraculous visions should cease; but when I awoke fully I found myself still lying in bed so that I had not really left my bed at all. *One should not ridicule the details given above about the items of food. The words used for these items of food are closely connected with the writing-down-system* which will be described later; they therefore demonstrate quite clearly the intention which prompted these dream visions.
>
> (Schreber, 1903/2000, p.71, n.37, italics added)

With notable clarity, Schreber explains that the words designating the foods have not been chosen at random, but are present because of their linguistic connection with what he calls the "writing-down-system", which he explains in detail in his *Memoirs*.

On this point, Lacan comments:

> You will notice that he introduces the dream as something that belongs essentially to the world of language. It isn't beside the point to observe the surprising illogicality that this represents on the part of an insane person who isn't supposed to be aware of the highly significant character that since Freud we give to dreams.
> (Lacan, 1955–56/1997, p.211)

On account of this quality of Schreber's relation to his dreams, we should say that he is a skilful reader, a skilful articulator of the signifier, both in its resonances within the dream narrative and in the words that name his everyday experience. Yet we must also note that, in his case, the supposition that his dreams are not his own, but instillations of a higher will, could constitute an obstacle to granting them their proper place within a treatment. Since Schreber did not have an analyst, we cannot know whether this might have been modified through a transferential encounter.

### 6.4 Dream Series

Another aspect emphasised by the authors mentioned above – treated in greater detail by Boukhabza, though it also appears in Apollon, Bergeron, and Cantin – and which we ourselves frequently encounter in clinical practice, is that dreams tend to become organised into series; series that revolve around certain themes and signifiers. In a manner akin to the 'continued story' observed by Freud (1923/1981, p.111), dreams display the successive elaboration of certain elements, which are taken up again and transformed during the course of the treatment; to the point that, as Boukhabza suggests, certain dreams may come to fulfil a quilting function, condensing several associative threads that run through the dream scene and the analysand's history.

In this respect, we could say that the functioning of dreams within the treatment is no different from what is found in neurotics. Through the testimonies of the pass, we are already familiar with the indexical function certain dreams acquire at the end of an analysis (Labaronnie, 2016; Mazzuca, 2011; Yacoi, 2002, 2012), and with the way in which dream series emerge from them – or become knotted to them – elaborating repetitive elements throughout the treatment. Following Boukhabza, we shall say that dreams situated in this way perform a function of naming *jouissance*. Their unfolding may be observed in case A. (Chapter 9).

In agreement with this author, we maintain that dream-work allows the exportation of *jouissance* towards *lalangue*, through a work of ciphering that follows the Freudian rules of displacement and condensation.

# 7 Dream-Work and *Jouissance*

With regard to *jouissance*, we propose that at least two processes are at play in dream-work. These could be ordered according to the coordinates set out by Lacan in *La troisième* (1975/2007):

1) the "taming" of *jouissance* through *lalangue* (p.35), by means of the activation of the resonances of language, which allow the mobilisation of the *jouissance* fixed in the body. Let us remember that Lacan redefines the drive as "the echo in the body of a fact of saying" (1975–76/2016, p.9). Since Freud, the drive has been defined as a concept on the frontier between the psychical and the bodily, and we cannot fail to note the bidirectional movements that make it a force both affected by and in turn affecting the act of saying. That which in the drives is *jouissance* can be worked upon by the machinery of *lalangue*, that is, by sounds, echoes, and homophonies.
2) the "precipitation" of *lalangue* in the letter (Lacan, 1975/2007, p.49): the passage from the continuous, the unrepresentable and the infinite, to the countable and finite dimension of the letter.

Dreams offer ample evidence of both operations. And in saying this we must think of *ciphering* and of *deciphering* together, since these ultimately constitute a single operation – provided that such deciphering leads not to a signification but to a character:

> And this is the only exorcism of which psychoanalysis is capable, it's because decipherment comes down to what is the character, to what is the symptom, it's something which above all does not stop

DOI: 10.4324/9781003755166-10

> writing itself in the real. And that setting out to tame it to the point where language can be ambiguous.
>
> (Lacan, 1975/2007, p.49)

The taming Lacan speaks of here is not located in a deciphering that leads to a meaning, but in one that leads to the character – to the letter in which equivocation plays – and which exorcises that *jouissance* which, through the very work of *lalangue*, has already been somewhat tamed.

With this key in mind, *The Interpretation of Dreams* could be revisited so as to extract from it the characters to which dreams lead – characters which Freud himself knew well how to isolate, even if they can be difficult to trace in that work, where they are immersed in a circuit of significations that confuse and divert. This is the case, for example, with the writing *mund*, contained in *Sigmund* and in the phrase "She would then have opened her mouth (*mund)* properly" (Freud, 1900/1971, p.111), from his paradigmatic dream.

Another interesting reflection on this topic can be found in *Radiophonie*,[1] where Lacan (1970) links displacement and condensation with passages from the real to the symbolic and vice versa, opening a hypothesis as to why the work with dreams can have such propitious effects – for any clinical structure. These ideas allow us to connect the mechanisms discovered by Freud with the distinction between registers proposed by Lacan.

Condensation, Lacan will say, allows for "the return of the impossible, to be conceived of as the limit by which the category of the real is installed by the symbolic" (Lacan, 1970, p.10). The notion of limit here is fundamental, for it is not a matter of our conceiving the real as inhabitable, but of being able to extract the clinical consequences of the inscription of a possible edge for the lawless real – an inscription in which the dream collaborates tirelessly. "I displace myself with the displacement of the real in the symbolic, and I condense myself to give weight to my symbols in the real, as suits tracking the unconscious (*comme il convient à suivre l'inconscient à la trace*)", Lacan says there (p.12). He therefore considers that a symbol arising from condensation carries real weight – an assertion not difficult to verify if we think of condensed signifiers – those of the Rat Man, for example – which, if graphically represented as a network (as Freud does in his Signorelli example (1901/2000)), can be read as nodal signifiers: centres of condensation of *jouissance* that knot and connect numerous associative lines. These are signifiers with weight in the real. Why? Because of what they condense – that is, because of the quantity of associative threads they gather, which in turn gives them another consistency at the level of *jouissance*: they become command centres of repetition. The real is defined there by always returning to the same place and also by constituting an unsymbolisable remainder.

The other operation, displacement, allows for a treatment of the real by way of the symbolic. The clearest example is that of mourning and traumatic experiences, after which there often follows a series of dreams that persistently attempt to symbolise the hole in the real reopened by the events. These dreams make full use of displacement, since they tend to present numerous variations on the same theme and transformations of the signifier that respond to the movement of affect from one to another. In that displacement, we may suppose, something of the affect is gradually worked through; it softens, as though at each step crumbs were being shed and left along the way. It is an operation of loss.

Both modalities are interwoven and often impossible to separate, since neither functions without the other. Their distinction nonetheless allows for the identification of basic clinical phenomena, amply demonstrated by the authors we have been discussing in their accounts of several cases of psychosis. Displacement serves particularly well to name what occurs when an analysand begins to recount their dreams, to listen to them, and to question them: something of the mortifying *jouissance* begins to be worked through by way of its linkage with successive signifiers, through the displacement from one element of the dream to another, but also from the dream towards memories and associations. The clinical effects of this work are well known to psychoanalysts: a certain relief quickly ensues.

Condensation, for its part, serves better to designate what Boukhabza (2012, 2013) remarks concerning the progression of the treatment to an advanced stage, where certain brief dreams come to name *jouissance* and to function as a knotting or quilting point. This can be clearly observed in the cases she reports, and it is also something noted in the clinic of the pass, since the testimonies abound with dreams of this kind, possessing a nominative value – minimal, highly condensed biographical dreams.

In order to name these operations, we believe that the terms *displacement* and *condensation* are preferable to those of *metonymy* and *metaphor*, which in linguistics do not carry exactly the same meaning

Lacan gave them and which, moreover, seem to refer solely to symbolic operations – substituting one signifier for another, for example – where it would be somewhat more difficult to locate the real at stake. In *Radiophonie*, Lacan (1970) speaks of displacement and condensation rather than metaphor and metonymy, at least when theorising the relation of the symbolic to the real. These terms also have the advantage of referring us to the question of the *treatment of affect*, so well delineated by Freud with regard to these mechanisms, and above all in relation to dreams.

Returning to the operations mentioned in *La troisième* (Lacan, 1975/2007), we may say that displacement belongs to the first – the taming of *jouissance* through the work of *lalangue* – and condensation to the second – the passage from *lalangue* to the letter, that littoral between the symbolic and the real, that inscriptional mark to which Lacan seems to allude when he speaks of 'giving weight to symbols in the real'.

## Note

1 Translator's note: No official English translation of "Radiophonie" (Lacan, 1970) exists. The translations of passages from this text used throughout are taken from Jack W. Stone's unpublished translation, available at [www.lacantokyo.org/img/Radiophonie_tr_en.pdf]. The original French text is published in Lacan, J. (2001). Autres écrits. Paris: Seuil.

# 8 Some Published Clinical Examples

Fortunately, the body of work published over the past few decades on the use of dreams in the treatment of psychoses has not been lacking in examples. Most of it comes from cases that are recounted at some length, whose dreams are reported and articulated in relation the progress of the treatment.

We shall return here to two of them, in order to offer the reader an approximate sense of what this literature contributes clinically.

## 8.1 The Case of M. Renard, by Danielle Bergeron

The Case of M. Renard, presented by Danielle Bergeron, abounds in examples of dreams, associations, and modifications in subjective position.

At the outset, this analysand brought dreams that were nothing more than chains of words, testifying to the intrusion of voices into his thinking: loose signifiers, decontextualised and without referent. The recounting of these dreams gave rise to few or no associations.

Gradually, the analyst reports, the dreams began to refer back to scenes from his history, especially to scenes of aggression directed towards him – initially on the part of his mother, but also by many others at different moments in his life. A history thus began to take shape that was new for him, one in which he was able to account for experiences of rejection by others, which he attributed to his physical appearance and to his shyness. The work with his dreams also made it possible to put into words persistent feelings of impotence in relation to women, alternating with repeated heartbreaks and feelings of nullification in the face of the other's mockery.

DOI: 10.4324/9781003755166-11

Throughout the treatment, the work with dreams did not rely on what the analyst might hear or the interpretations she might attempt, but on what the analysand himself was capable of saying and concluding for his everyday life. In this way, genuine analytic work gradually supplanted the work of delusion. Dreams of a different nature began to appear, such as the following: "I thought I was going to pilot an American fighter jet, an F-18, in Star Wars and engage in combat. In the back, there was a square wooden box, empty" (Bergeron, 2008, p.233). The analysand associates the empty box with the coffin that awaits him when he dies, and goes on to speak about the suicide of a French writer. The analyst points out that he is very often drawn to authors who have written or reflected on death, or who have taken their own lives. This intervention allows the analysand to speak about an issue that has accompanied him since childhood: his life is a constant struggle against death. He even recalls, with anguish, having burst into tears at the age of six upon realising that he would one day die.

When M. Renard began his analysis, the voices ridiculed and threatened him, making particularly humiliating remarks about his penis and, at times, about his face. This was the period in which the dreams took up loose, hallucinatory signifiers. When the treatment had progressed, this analysand reported noticing that the work of the unconscious quietened the voices. By that point, the voices had ceased to intervene during the sessions, but they still tormented him in certain public spaces, especially in grocery shops. He expressed the wish for these voices to disappear, yet also acknowledged that at times he wanted to preserve them, since he felt very lonely. In saying this, he became aware that the voices intensified when he spent more than two or three hours alone in his bed, after which he decided to begin avoiding such prolonged moments of isolation.

Furthermore, in the treatment of this psychotic analysand, a series of dreams takes up the theme of exhibitionism and gradually works through it, with increasing possibilities of offering the dreamer the coordinates of his position as object. As the analysis progresses, the dreams become clearer in this respect: they begin to show scenes in which he appears naked before the gaze of others, at times on the verge of masturbating, or else represented within a group of "submissive men" (Bergeron, 2008, p.234), and among young men who display their penis in inappropriate situations. These dreams lead M. Renard to reconsider a series of lived situations in which he finds himself in a passive position: initially in relation to a cousin who humiliated him from an early age, and later in his workplace – where he eventually manages to take a stand in situations he considers unjust. At the same time, he is led to question certain exhibitionistic habits he himself had practised and which in some cases placed him at risk of a legal sanction. At a certain point, after working through several dreams bordering on this theme, he decides to stop posing as a nude model in art classes, since he no longer wishes to exhibit his body. Simultaneously, he dares to make a brief remark when a customer mistreats an elderly woman in front of him, and in a session states that he has begun to feel more at ease in his body.

> At this point in the treatment, through dreams that he still struggled to associate with most of the time, a scene came to light: one from when he was five years old, when a doctor examined him, handling him, while his mother watched him suffer and laughed at him, as though mocking his genitals in danger. This scene had taken root at the core of a repetition whose origin he was progressively learning to recognise, while in the analysis, knowledge was being constructed about some of his behaviours and attitudes towards women.
>
> (Bergeron, 2008, p.236)

Other dreams later come to inscribe something the analysand regards as an indication concerning the subjective position he must attain. "I am speaking about a film in a discussion group. Johnny is there, blond, slim, seductive. I think that he has sex with the girls. I envy him", says this analysand (Bergeron, 2008, p.246). Despite always complaining about his bad luck with women, on this occasion he associates the dream with a text by Bertrand Russell, in which it is mentioned that a peacock should not grieve because another peacock has a more beautiful tail. He concludes that if a peacock with magnificent plumage, with beautiful colours, envies another peacock, this only brings hatred and jealousy. These reflections on the dream lead him to consider that the issue is "to be happy with one's own means, with what one is" (p.247).

Shortly thereafter, he recounts a dream in which a man he respects advises him: "Stop being ashamed – be a man!" (p.247). All of this is also articulated with a symptomisation of his obesity and excessive eating, which is gradually transformed as the dreams bring into play – and make it possible to put into words – the coordinates and effects of his bingeing, linking them to the difficulties connected with his body image. Throughout this trajectory, there remains a persistent fear that others might be able to guess his thoughts – a delusional idea that runs through the entire material and is interwoven quite naturally with the content of his dreams and his associations. We find here once again the fact observed by Freud: that the analysis of a dream may distill an obsessional idea, a hysterical idea, or a delusional idea as its preconscious motive. What is interesting to note is how this delusional fear permeates the material and becomes woven into the dreams in such a way that it ceases to constitute a certainty and instead comes to be named as a fear, as a recurrent idea that torments him and gives rise to certain thoughts and certain acts.

## 8.2 The Case of A., by Dominique Boukhabza

Regarding the analysand A., we have already mentioned the "dream of the voices", in which he progressively removes bugs from his ears and then wakes up. This dream corresponds to a period of the treatment during which A. had just been hospitalised, which the analyst attributes to a decompensation linked to the establishment of the transference. This effect of the beginning of analysis in psychotics – formerly problematised, and which led to the discouragement of properly analytic work with material such as dreams – is currently defended by the analysts we have been discussing. In their view, such crises would in any case have been triggered, and constitute a lesser evil provided arrangements are in place to accompany the course of these episodes. These crises should not be feared, they argue, since they consider them the turbulent passage through a period that subsequently makes analysis possible.

A., returns from hospitalisation to seek out his analyst and recounts this dream – in which he removes the bugs from his ears – thereby verbalising his request explicitly: "The voices, I would like them to stop" (p.186).

It was also in relation to this analysand that we mentioned the author's hypothesis that the series formed by dreams throughout the treatment converge upon a pivotal dream, which she does not hesitate to regard as a quilting point – a form of knotting, for those who wish to invoke the Lacan of the knots. Over the ten years of analysis she conducted with A., Boukhabza noted down the dreams at the end of each session. At the time she had no idea of the meaning this material would later acquire, yet she felt the need to transcribe and preserve it, since it seemed to her to be valuable material.

When she began to study these notes some years later, she observed, for example, that A.'s associations had progressively increased as the analysis advanced. Day residues, by contrast, were never evoked.

One of the series into which, for the analyst, this patient's dreams are organised revolves around study; she calls them "study dreams" (Boukhabza, 2012, p.19). These are dreams presenting him in situations involving the pursuit of studies – a task the patient had abandoned after his father's death and whose completion had been his father's wish. The analysand considers that continuing his studies would have given him access to the world of work and to marriage, yet declares that he has always detested writing, particularly because of certain dictation exercises his mother forced him to do at home, for which she would slap him if they were not carried out correctly.

At times, when the academic year began again at a school near his adult home, A. would start to hear voices once more – voices of children or young girls saying "*calandair*", a neologism he associates with "calendar, periods, young girls". The onset of the voices is situated around an encounter with a waitress in a bar, a very beautiful young woman who makes a strong impression on him. He has the impression that she went straight up to him and said something close to "I love you" directly to his face, though not exactly that – the sound she uttered was very similar to his own first name. This young woman visits him at home and he cooks for her. On some occasions they have sex, a situation he describes as one rather initiated by her, while he simply allows himself to be acted upon.

A. frequently links children with women: "children and women are complementary" (p.16), he says. The voices he hears – always children's voices, generally without clear words – thus become connected with the triggering conjuncture: the encounter with a woman.

With regard to the voices, just as with his "study dreams", A. states: "they excite me" (p.20). In one of his dreams, the analyst is a governess and A. is one of the pupils in her class.

Another series is constituted by the "hole dreams" (p.20), which take up the term *trou* (hole). In different dreams, he either makes holes or finds holes in objects or in his own body. Finally, he dreams that during an operation his heart – the organ whose failure had caused his father's death – is replaced; he is given a new heart that allows him to breathe, walk, and run. A. recalls that he was the one who used to assist his father when the latter could not breathe during his illness. He dreams that his father runs, falls, begins to suffocate, and that he lifts him up.

A third series is that of the "cutting dreams", in which A. takes part in fights and is wounded – sometimes himself, at other times others (friends, for example). Many of these dreams bring his ears onto the scene, though from a different angle from that of the voices that afflict him there. In one, his ears are the site of a swelling that spreads to his cheeks; in another, he receives a cut near an ear. In a further dream, he is cut during a fight, yet no blood flows from the wounds – unlike what occurred in his "hole dreams", where blood did emerge – and A. says to himself, "this will scar on its own" (p.21). No analyst, I believe, would fail to hear in these dreams a changing relation to castration. In another dream, it is a hook that cuts him – lodged in his body yet causing no harm; indeed, in the dream he himself inserts and removes it. The hook leads him to associate with the fishing trips he used to take with his father and with the fish, his father's zodiac sign. The analyst also notes that *hameçon* (hook), in French, sounds like *âme-son* (soul-sound). This is what he plunged in and withdrew at will, something that remained embedded in without causing pain, an element he moreover associates with his father.

A fourth series revolves around the eyebrows. The analyst recounts the two most significant dreams:

> My grandfather looks at me. He says: you have forgotten something. I say: Ah, yes, the circumflex accent is missing. I draw a circumflex accent beneath the eyebrows. This sequence could evoke the expression 'eyebrows in the shape of a circumflex accent', but this is not mentioned by A. [...] Here again, it is a matter of a mark on the body – this time, the grandfather's body.
>
> (p.22)

What is at stake here is that which frames the gaze: eyebrows arched in a certain way, recalling the stroke of a linguistic element such as the circumflex accent. As Boukhabza remarks, this mark on the body borrows the form of a graphic stroke of the letter.

Shortly afterwards, a very brief dream takes up and connects several of these elements:

> 'I have blood in my eyebrows'. This dream is then associated with a childhood memory. As a child, he wore a dressing on his face for many years. He appears like this in the photographs taken by his father, who loved taking photographs. The dressing was in fact a bandage to protect his forehead. At that time in his childhood, which he dates to around the age of five, he would frequently fall and injure his forehead. His mother used to say that his face was too heavy.
>
> (p.22)

On the basis of these dreams, A. says that he begins to notice that words take on a "personal", "physical" meaning – that they "take on a body" (p.22). He responds with a series of dreams that leave him thinking: "I have a child in my arms. I am the father; it is a newborn. Yet it speaks …"; "I am also that child"; "I always dream about my studies …, but now I succeed" (p.23). In this context, he stops smoking.

Subsequently, certain dreams return to the theme of giving up cigarettes and connect it with the theme of the hole, the face, and the falls he used to have as a child.

The hypothesis proposed by Boukhabza is that, here, dreams are equivalent to associative chains.

> As we have said, associations do exist, but they are infrequent. We put forward the hypothesis that the missing associations must be sought in the content of subsequent dreams.
>
> It is indeed revealed that dreams follow certain threads. They seem to regroup into series, either by taking up the same theme (studies, fights, the father's death …), or by organising themselves around a particular element (hole, cut …). Certain dreams lie at the point of convergence of two series (the dream of the circumflex accent, the dream of the crown). [...]
>
> We are thus led to the following hypothesis: the continuation of dreams would come to knot together an interrupted signifying chain; the work of writing and then of reading the dream within the transference would allow for an articulation of elements that had until then remained isolated, as well as the production of meanings that had hitherto been absent.
>
> (pp.24–25)

Following these ideas, the author explains that, in her view, the dream-work made it possible in this treatment to re-knot the Real, the Symbolic, and the Imaginary, and that the installation of the Other scene – that of the dream – enabled an operation upon *jouissance*, a kind of emptying that brought about the extinction of the voices.

# 9 The Case of C.

## 9.1 The Clinical Picture

The treatment I am about to present began within the framework of the care provided to students at the National University of La Plata by the Health Service of the Rectorate.

At the outset, the consultation was presented as motivated by conflicts in cohabitation and by certain physical symptoms that I shall detail later.

The patient, whom I shall call C., is twenty-seven years old and is studying for a degree related to early childhood. After passing, with great difficulty, several subjects in another course of study, she enrolled in this second programme, where her progress has likewise been far from smooth.

Initially reticent and sparing in her speech, she gradually begins to recount what has brought her to consult. She lives with her brother and his girlfriend in an atmosphere of visible hostility, marked by shouting, mutual insults, and accusations. C. does not locate the source of these affronts in her relationship with her brother, but in the involvement of the third party in the discord – his girlfriend, whom she will never call by name. "This person", as she refers to her, possesses in her account all the characteristics of a usurper: she lives there by favour, creates conflicts, and carries out small actions intended to irritate her, such as moving an object a few centimetres to make it more difficult for her to pass along the corridor of the apartment, or occupying the entire drying rack so as to leave no space for C.'s laundry.

During the first months of treatment, the quarrels do not cease, and on each occasion her physical sufferings worsen: stomach pains, a feeling of suffocation, pain in the chest. All the physicians she has

DOI: 10.4324/9781003755166-12

consulted point towards a "nervous" aetiology, a hypothesis C. herself shares.

Her brother and his girlfriend are likewise uncomfortable with this cohabitation. It is they who inform the parents that the atmosphere has become unbearable and that they do not know how to achieve any tranquillity with C. Following an episode that ends in a violent confrontation with her brother, her parents travel from their city of residence and attempt to intervene. The mother devotes herself to calming her for several days, taking walks with her and asking her to cooperate so that there may be fewer disturbances. The father, for the first and only time, admits that he does not know what to do and asks that they try to get along.

Weeping inconsolably, C. tells me that during the parents' visit her brother and "this person" accused her of having done certain things – things that she herself had previously told me: removing their clothes from the drying rack, playing music at full volume on Saturday mornings so that they could not sleep late, shouting at them because they do not clean, and similar actions. Only that, in her account, these behaviours were logical and beyond reproach, as well as entirely devoid of malice. For her brother, by contrast – at least as she relates it – such behaviours are arbitrary and excessive impositions. Indeed, from the way she recounts it, it is not difficult to imagine that C.'s actions, her constant control over the order and cleanliness of the apartment and over the schedules she considers should be adopted by everyone, resemble the obligations and prohibitions of a totalitarian regime.

There is no room for doubt in her; her discourse presents no fissures through which the possibility of putting herself in the other's shoes might emerge. Any intervention aimed at slightly limiting her demands falls on deaf ears.

Her anguish, moreover, continues to increase; the accusations have left her exhausted and without the will to do anything for days. She feels unjustly blamed and is desperate to obtain justice. Only one intervention manages to give some lodging to her anguish: I tell her that we all have people who criticise what we do, that this is not a serious matter, and that although her version of events may not be compatible with theirs, this is not something she cannot live with. This produces a noticeable relief and ushers in a phase in which she "plays down" – such is her expression – these differences.

It is worth noting that throughout this entire period, from the very beginning of the treatment, C. never once contemplated the possibility of ending this cohabitation, nor even of speaking with her parents about other possible options, since what would be right, in her view, would be for "this person" to leave.

The detail that, from the very first moment, made her sister-in-law deserving of her suspicion is striking: like all the partners her brothers and sisters have had, "this person" entered the parental home as a visitor and went straight into the living room without greeting the father – after which he took against her, as he had done with each and every one of his sons-in-law and daughters-in-law, and for the same reason. Despite this account, C. also maintains that the father allows and defends "this person" living with them in this apartment, which he purchased with great effort so that they might come to study. The reason, according to her, is that the father knows "this person's" family and does not wish to fall out with anyone. Thus, the supposed rejection on the father's part towards "this person" has been transferred onto C., and has taken root in her for years.

In addition to this brother, C. has an older sister – who recently became a mother – a younger brother, and a half-brother, conceived by the father in an extramarital relationship, who from a certain age lived with them, only to leave upon turning eighteen and never again make contact with any member of the family. This half-brother was also the object of C.'s hatred from the moment he appeared in their lives, although at present they have no news of him.

## 9.2 A Place for C.

The year before C. was born, her mother gave birth to a girl who died after only a few months of life as a result of respiratory problems: "she suffocated", C. says. The family narrative recounts that C. herself also came close to dying during childbirth, and for the same reason: lack of air.

Like Salvador Dalí, C. has no proper name of her own: both her first and second names are those that had already been given to this deceased sister.

With this account, it becomes apparent that the hostility towards her sister-in-law is not her only reason for consulting. She is deeply moved when she decides to tell me that, at night, three very sad thoughts come to her. One concerns this deceased sister and the conclusion she has reached: that had this death not occurred, she herself would not be in the world. C. is in this sister's place, usurping her position – this is a certainty for her. Since she has a younger brother, on one occasion I point out that if her sister had not died, as she maintains, and given that her parents continued to have children, perhaps she would indeed be in the world, but she would have a different name. I am not sure whether this intervention produced any effect, yet the question of the name will be taken up again (see Section 9.6.8).

The second thought that torments her is that her mother has told her about the asphyxia she suffered at birth, which left her on the brink of death. She thinks about that near-death, and becomes anguished.

The third thought is that, when she was less than a year old, her parents decided to entrust her to a family of friends to be raised, citing financial difficulties and the fact that her brother – the one with whom she now lives – did not want her. According to her mother's account, this arrangement lasted a week or perhaps a month, after which C. returned to her family "because she cried". Her history thus situates her as lacking a proper name and, for the second time, as having been rejected.

Many months later she will tell me that, when she visits them, her father constantly alludes to this deceased sister. He says things such as, "Just imagine if, instead of you being here, your sister were here – what she would have been like", or "She would surely do well at university". On that occasion, with the transference already established, I expressed my opposition to these remarks and to the continuation of a discourse that makes of her a mere substitute for her sister. Subsequently, I have been able to think that this, together with the question – which I introduced at that moment – of whether she had ever considered changing her name, or choosing a name that would be hers alone, marked a decisive turning point in the treatment.

## 9.3 The Social Bond

At the time she began treatment, C. had no female friends and never had. She did, however, have two male friends she had never met in person and had come to know through an online chat. She converses with them very often via chat, and they are the ones who encourage her to carry on when she loses all desire to live.

Nor has she had a partner or sexual relations. The closest she has come was a five-year relationship with a young man from a northern province, whom she also met through chat and has never seen in person. They communicate every day, in exchanges marked by both intense arguments and moments of mutual support. She has already wished to meet him on several occasions, yet each time he has stood her up just as she was preparing to travel to a city halfway between them.

To what does she attribute her lack of friends throughout school and university? "To distrust", she says, and is unable to explain much further. For her, the social bond is either familial – laden with torment – or virtual, sustained through online chats. This begins to change during the treatment, as she starts to form some connections and no longer reports problems of distrust, nor do delusional interpretations arise as they did regarding her sister-in-law.

From a certain point onwards, she notices that one of the things that alleviates her stomach pain is leaving the house. With this in mind, she makes an effort to create some social ties herself, especially with girls from the student union, who eventually invite her to join. This inaugurates a new chapter in which she shares *mate* with two or three friends, attends a few very occasional evening outings, and above all takes part in meetings related to student union activities. She gets on very well with these people – they help her with her exams and serve as a refuge when she needs to get out of the house. Her virtual friends continue to play a significant role: when she is truly unwell, they are the ones who have the right words to lift her spirits.

## 9.4 A Name for Her Suffering

As the interviews progressed, and guided by the dreams I will detail later, I was able to locate a signifier that I consider central and orienting for the transference. It does not concern any elementary phenomenon, for C. suffers only from certain delusional interpretations circumscribed to the rivalry with her sister-in-law, and presents neither florid delusions nor hallucinations. Her relationship with her body is deeply afflicted, yet it does not manifest through any form of disintegration; rather, one might say that she becomes aware of her body through the fact that she suffers pains: principally in the stomach, but also in the chest and with a lack of air at the most severe moments – which recalls both her near-death by asphyxia at birth and the cause of her sister's death.

What I ultimately identify as central is, in her own words, a "falling". Several issues are condensed there. On the one hand, her recurrent dreams prior to the treatment. On the other, and very markedly, a certain melancholic affect, when she feels the lack of love from her family – "I have never felt what it is to be loved by someone", she will say – or when she thinks she will not be able to succeed in her studies. At times, she falls because she cannot find a place in the Other; on certain days she explicitly wonders what she has come into the world for. Her relationship to her studies follows the rhythm of these falls in mood and interest, alternating with days of greater activity and renewed vitality.

When this aspect of her suffering begins to be spoken about in analysis, the quarrels with her sister-in-law and brother progressively diminish, until they disappear altogether; to such an extent that, several months later, I ask her whether she still lives with them. Surprisingly, she replies that her brother has returned to their hometown and that she is now living with "this person", without speaking to one another, yet also without altercations. By that time, she frequently makes use of a phrase that I had taken from her discourse at a certain moment: "to play it down". With this resource, she manages to navigate many situations that previously would have ended in disaster.

At times, the "falling" also takes hold of the body: when she is very worried about examinations, afraid that she will not be able to continue her course of study and will have to choose another path, she feels pain in her chest, lack of air, and occasionally a weakness she interprets as a drop in blood pressure, especially upon getting up in the morning.

The friends who know her best encourage her to carry on, telling her that she can manage, that she must not let herself fall. They are her friends from the chat, those who know so well what, in her case, constitutes that "disturbance that occurred at the inmost juncture of the subject's sense of life" (Lacan, 1959/2005, p.559).

Thus, when I ask her whether she has thought about how to proceed once her treatment at the Rectorate Health Service comes to an end, she replies that if there is any possibility of continuing with me elsewhere, she would accept, because she has been thinking: "if I stop coming here, I will fall". Some time later, I begin to see her in my private consulting room. To my surprise, she tells me that she was already familiar with it, since I myself had received her there on a day when we found the Rectorate closed and she needed to talk. I had no recollection of this.

### 9.5 Literality

In time, C. also tells me about a certain sensitivity she has to words, both for better and for worse. Her gastroenterologist, for example, once made the mistake of remarking, quite in passing, that a relative had been forced to abandon a university degree because of symptoms similar to hers. We were able to arrive at this remark – and to question its universality, much to her relief – only after several sessions in which she appeared extremely nervous, with intensified pains and a more marked despondency, yet without being able to identify the reason. It was only when she recalled that conversation that we were able to detach her from the bleak destiny to which that utterance had left her bound.

In the same way, she finds considerable support in the lyrics of certain songs, especially those by Andrés Calamaro. Simply by playing a track in which he sings "no te preocupes, Paloma" ("don't worry, Paloma"), she stops worrying. Yet these songs also have another use: "I begin to understand; they help me understand what is happening to me". Once this use is articulated within the transference, it becomes more frequent and clearly established as a resource for her. Thus, at a moment of rupture with her virtual partner – with whom she repeatedly breaks up and reconciles – she listened to a song that said: "tu amor no es mi enfermedad, es sólo un espacio vacío"[1] ("your love is not my illness, it is only an empty space"), and this calmed her; she understood it to mean "that feelings may exist, but that if things don't work out, one must let go". Similarly, the lyrics of another band, which say "quiero que me trates suavemente" ("I want you to treat me gently"), prompt her to demand better treatment from the young man, who often becomes enraged and insults her through chat. There is also a song that calms her when she worries about things she sees on the news, titled "Estadio azteca". She explains: "It made me think about why I was here, in the world. I didn't feel that I belonged, that I had a reason to be here. Whether I am meant to be here, or whether she should be here instead".

With the exception of the gastroenterologist's remark, this adhesive relation to lyrics tends to work more in her favour than against her. Evidently, there is some degree of choice on her part regarding what she listens to.

When the question of what is "hers" begins to become established within the transference – through dreams, and through a reconsideration of her proper name and her place in the world – she buys herself a guitar. She tells me this only after having done so, and points out that it was the first time she had ever bought something for herself. She is enthusiastic about learning to play her favourite songs, an activity to which she devotes herself by watching tutorials on the internet.

## 9.6 Dreams

### *9.6.1 Two Recurrent Dreams*

In one of the first interviews, I asked C. whether she dreams. She replied that she does, and that she has certain recurrent dreams in particular. In one of them, she falls endlessly, in the midst of total darkness. She does not wake up immediately; rather, the falling lasts for a certain length of time.

The other recurrent dream is as follows: she is in the midst of darkness, unable to see anything, and with her hands she searches for something to cling to; she cries out, yet finds nothing.

From the outset, these recurrent dreams situate us in relation to a *falling* – all the more striking in that it does not immediately provoke awakening, leaving the dreamer in a continuous feeling of descent. Dreams of falling are considered typical (Freud, 1900/1971, p.241), yet it is more usual to wake at once when the fall occurs. The infinitisation of this fall in C. cannot but surprise us. Taken metaphorically, it leads us to think of her lack of a place in the primordial Other – the place from which she falls – and of her struggle to carve out a place of her own. From that point onwards, C. begins to recount the dreams she has throughout the treatment.

### *9.6.2 First Dream*

"I was arguing with my brother in the apartment. He was telling me that I was always the one who started the arguments and that I had nothing to do there, that I should not interfere".

This dream, which occurred within the context of the first interviews – when hostility in the shared living arrangement was the central theme of her consultation – already presented two key elements: C.'s sense of having no place in the world – "I had nothing to do there" – and the outline of a subjective rectification – "that I was always the one who started the arguments and that I should not interfere". Both aspects appear disguised within a scene of quarrelling, the first point intermingled with the other statements for greater concealment. I recall asking her what she thought about what the dream was saying – about the idea that she started all the arguments and should not interfere. As a good paranoiac, her incorrigible condition allowed her to ignore these assertions completely – even though they were included in her own dream! – and, of course, I did not insist. The rectification introduced by the dream is firmly rejected; for her, it is simply an accusation. We shall return to this outline of rectification in the final section.

Let us note, from the outset, that all the dreams C. has brought to her analysis thus far are nightmares – scenes that torment her and which she recounts as a way of taking distance from them. Once narrated, there are very few elements she can associate with. Yet it is evident that she needs to tell them to me. One might say that the analyst assumes there the function Lacan termed that of *dépotoir*, a *rubbish dump* (1955–56/1997, p.39). C. puts them into words and, in doing so, experiences relief. The analyst, however, need not be satisfied with this alone. As we shall see, at certain moments I make some remarks. My aim is not to decipher these dreams, but rather to extract from them a wisp of desire – a life-giving pathway capable of countering the drift towards melancholisation.

### *9.6.3 Second Dream*

"There were many cats around a swimming pool. An injured cat appeared; it was missing a paw. I was shouting, 'It's dying on me, it's dying on me' (*Se me muere, se me muere*[2]).

This dream occurred shortly after the interviews had begun. C. had already told me about the thoughts that come to her at night, yet her everyday concern remained centred on the problems of cohabitation. Nevertheless, it is easy to perceive that this dream brings onto the scene a possible version of the words someone might have uttered at the moment of her birth, when the asphyxia threatened to kill her: "it's dying on me, it's dying on me". This is, in fact, what happened to her sister. I do not make this explicit, but I do ask about the swimming pool and the cats. Concerning the former, she tells me that it resembles the one at a house where her mother works as a domestic employee. The lady of the house is a journalist, and her husband is a painter. On this point, she adds no further details.

As for the cats, by contrast, she has much to say. Not only are they her favourite pets, but they are also objects of her solidarity: for several years she has been involved in what is known as "cat fostering", providing shelter, food, and treatment for abandoned cats and kittens. This activity keeps her in contact with other people, who contribute money, medicines, and food, and help to find homes for the cats once they have recovered. This vocation will become the subject of several conversations throughout the treatment. At first, the presence of cats in her bedroom was also a source of conflict with her brother and "this person", but she did not allow herself to be intimidated and always defended this activity, which she finds deeply engaging.

The cat's missing paw, besides evoking for me the Lacanian theory of a missing element in psychosis, also brings to mind once again Salvador Dalí, with those curious supporting crutches he placed beneath the objects in his paintings, thereby highlighting the absent support. As we can see, many of the associations C.'s dreams evoke in me remain within my own inner dialogue – a fact also noted by Cantin (2008), and which we referred to in Section 6.3.

Moreover, we should not lose sight of the fact that the opportunity to speak about the cats and about what they mean to her arises from this dream.

### *9.6.4 Third Dream*

C. tells me that it sometimes happens that she wakes up crying and continues to cry once awake, even though she does not always remember what she has dreamt. In this way, she attests to the very common continuity between dream and waking life that we have previously discussed. This is precisely what occurred following the next dream:

> I was arguing with my father and my mother; I was telling everyone to go to hell. I said, 'go to hell, all of you', and I left.

After recounting this dream, she adds the following: a few days earlier, during a telephone conversation in which she was voicing all her complaints about her brother and "this person", her mother had surprised her with the response: "well, I've had enough". Even more surprising is that, in that same week, she received an ultimatum from her virtual boyfriend on account of her negativity. "I'd rather distance myself", he said – a distance that, as I mentioned at the outset, would not last long, since their relationship is marked by repeated comings and goings.

Up to the moment of this dream, I was unaware of the existence of this virtual relationship or of her long-distance friends. The opportunity thus arose to speak for the first time about her relations with people outside the family and about the trait she termed "distrust", which makes social bonds difficult for her. Up to this point, her dreams serve to open up topics of conversation and to allow for historisation; from this account, for example, emerges the history of her distrust during her years at school.

Moreover, we can see that in the dream she introduces a cut, just as in reality her boyfriend and her mother had done. In this sense, the dream anticipates reality, revealing her desire, for the cut with that which causes her distress will begin with her decision to "play down" the actions of "this person" and of her brother. That "telling everyone to go to hell" displayed in the dream will come about later, and in a rather more peaceful manner, when she decides not to involve herself in certain arguments and, above all, not to remain listening to her father when he compares her with her deceased sister.

We might say of this dream what Freud observed: "*The ancient belief that dreams foretell the future is not wholly devoid of truth. By picturing our wishes as fulfilled, dreams are after all leading us into the future*" (1900/1971, p.621). And yet, as Freud goes on to express in the paragraph that follows, this future is closely bound to the past, and it is from there that it has been summoned to form part of the dream. We understand this as referring to something that has already occurred in C.'s life – a certain subtle cut that has probably already taken place – and of which the dream bears witness. If the future is to be awaited, it will be so that this cut may come to be recognised in new ways.

### *9.6.5 Fourth, Fifth, and Sixth Dreams*

"I had a serious illness; I was in a place with a dark background, and I was trying to get out of there. I didn't know where to go. Sometimes I let that happen".

I ask what she means by this. She explains that, at times, within these dreams of darkness she gives up and allows herself to be trapped by the dark; she abandons herself there. She immediately goes on to recount:

> Last week I dreamt that my teeth were falling out; they hurt and they fall out. They had never fallen out before, but last week one did fall out. I looked at it and it wasn't a molar … like a fresh one; it was from a long time ago, with pores. I was holding it in my hand and it was breaking. As if decalcified. Before, I had only dreamt that they were loose.

We might say that there is a convergence between the cut borne witness to in the third dream and this cut, which occurs for the first time in her recurrent dreams, where a calcified tooth finally falls out. A dream regarded as *typical* (Freud, 1900/1971, p.241), we see that it also appears in psychotic patients. In this case, it signals a change in relation to earlier dreams: the teeth that had formerly been loose now fall out. And what of that porous quality? Freud taught us that the dreamer is distributed among all the characters – and objects – of the dream. That tooth which falls out is, to some extent, herself, because she too has become porous, permeable, pierced through. This becomes perceptible in the transference.

I would like to introduce two remarks here. The first is that, according to my notes, the period of these dreams corresponds to her initial contacts with female classmates at the university who were involved in the student union. When she mentioned them, I would ask her to tell me something about them and about the relationship they were beginning to build.

The second remark is that each dream offered C. an opportunity to recount numerous events from her everyday reality, and for me, these dreams brought important information, allowing me to guide my questions, generally oriented towards learning more about her daily life, and thus to locate both her symptomatic aspects and her resources in the face of the invasive *jouissance* of an ever-incipient melancholisation. Unfortunately, the finer details of our conversations arising from each dream cannot be reconstructed. As always occurs when reviewing the notes and the recollections the analyst has been able to preserve, one is subjected to inevitable overlaps, to movements that become confused or merge at key points in the treatment, without it being possible to offer greater detail regarding the precise order of events.

Nonetheless, I hope that the reader can appreciate the interplay between the case data narrated at the outset and the texture of dreams that C. went on to recount. The correspondences are numerous, and her dream-life has undoubtedly borne witness to the movements and key points of this phase of the analysis.

After recounting the dream of the tooth falling out, C. comments: "it always happens to me that they are dreams that only show a certain moment; they don't have much development".

This remark surprises me and, moreover, gives rise to an intimate feeling of having been heard in what I did not say. C. has perceived very clearly my interest in dreams – material which habitually allows me to sustain my interest in those whose treatment is entrusted to me. Always having within reach a little well-polished desire, Lacan recommended to analysts (1960–61/2009, p.371). Each analyst, I assume, knows how to make clinical use of whatever most closely binds them to the possibility of analysing – and of not losing that desire which everyday life sometimes threatens. Thus, C.'s lament at not having dreams with greater development produces in me an intimate sensation of "touché!".

Perhaps it is in this encounter of desires that an analytic bond has been sustained; one that has not borne the marks of that paranoiac tendency she so readily recognises in herself: distrust.

In that same session, C. recounts another dream, which had occurred weeks earlier:

> There were some superheroes (this amuses her somewhat); one was Iron Man or Superman, he had a cape and a body of steel. The other was dressed entirely in black. They began to fight. I was watching. I didn't know where to put myself. I was looking for a place.

Once again, the theme of place emerges: where is the subject to find a place for herself? We shall see that her dreams return to this. The hostility of the environment, the fights, are also repeated; and this time the darkness of the void is replaced by the black attire of a superhero. I have not mentioned it previously, but the constant fighting is a feature of C.'s family of origin, and not only of her current living situation. Her father – a stern and demanding man, harsh in his words and strongly inclined to reproach – gradually corroded his relationship with each of his children. His wife, although she remains with him, has, according to C., never felt at ease nor expressed any affection for him. When C. visits her parental home, she suffers considerably and her mood deteriorates.

This dream also contains two details that merit mention. On the one hand, the presence of a drive-related activity: I was there, *watching*. On the other, the relation to knowledge. It is no longer a matter of her having *nothing to do there*, but rather of her *not knowing* where to put herself. She has already been told not to interfere, in another dream; yet here her *not-knowing* appears more clearly marked, which is quite a novelty for someone whose certainty of knowing – regarding the bad intentions of the Other – has been the very motive for consultation. The course of the analysis, for her as well, inaugurates a *not-knowing* that will prove fruitful.

### *9.6.6 Seventh Dream*

> It was about an argument with my family, in a desert. My mother was there, in a tent. I woke up crying. I was telling my father that I am a woman and that he was making a sexist distinction.

Here, once again, the crying from the dream continues into waking life.

One might say that the boundlessness of the darkness is replaced by a desert – which is not entirely boundless, insofar as the edges of the tent are present there. The tent is a place: a place in the midst of the desert. I do not recall whether I said anything about this during the session, or whether I simply thought it. She links the desert with a book she is reading, *The Alchemist*. We speak briefly about it.

This reference to her femininity also deserves our attention, as she had never previously commented on it, nor had she mentioned these "sexist distinctions". It should be noted that this dream is recounted after telling me that she had met with girls from the student union and that she was getting to know people. "Nice people – it's as if they already knew me", a phrase that is surprising coming from someone so distrustful. As part of the union, she takes part in activist activities involving the defence of students' rights and joining forces for collective struggles, some of which stem from feminist slogans. Let us not forget, moreover, that after abandoning an initial course of study, she has chosen a profession linked to women and early childhood.

With these companions, she attends a night out for the first time and, later on, they invite her to a barbecue – which she does not attend. As for the night out, she says she enjoyed herself and felt comfortable with the people she knew. Nevertheless, she drinks alcohol – also for the first time – and this produces in her a markedly sad disposition, leading her to end up crying and thinking about her most recent break-up with the young man she met online. When recounting this to me, she does so with a touch of laughter – more cheerful than dramatic – since the situation apparently led her into one or two embarrassing moments in front of her peers; something that does not mortify her in the least.

In the following session, she wants to tell me about a sensation she had during the week – something new which, evidently, has made an impression on her. "I was walking along, I saw babies, and I found myself wondering whether one day I might come to have that image within me". She explains that she is referring to becoming pregnant, to whether she might be able to be a mother. According to her account, she had not thought about this before; it is rather a new desire. It also frightens her, as she is not up to date with her gynaecological check-ups, and the last time she sought consultation she was advised to undergo tests, as she suffers from amenorrhoea. At no point does she allude to the matter of sexual relations as being necessary in order to conceive a child in the future (it is true that nowadays they are not necessarily so); indeed, at one point I ask her whether a man is required for that, and she replies that no, that she does not consider it necessary.

### *9.6.7 Eighth Dream*

After the summer break, we resume the sessions. In the first, she recounts the following: "today I woke up feeling afraid and startled. I'm walking down the street and it's as if there were no one there – it's like a void. I think, 'what am I doing here?'".

She has spent the summer at her parents' house. I notice her to be worse – sad, worried, nervous. It is the state that habitually follows each visit to her hometown. But this time, given that it was a prolonged stay, she seems worse than usual.

The following week, she recounts a nightmare:

> I've been having dreams of escaping from something, of being pursued. I was going to a party with classmates from high school

> and university. It was in a large building. I was sad, and they had invited me because of that. I decide to leave. I go down a long corridor; it was like a hospital. Some nurses with scrubs stop me; they tell me, 'you can't go through here', towards another corridor that was there. I arrive at a place where there were stretchers with many dismembered bodies. There was another corridor and a slide. I fell down it and couldn't get back up. I fell into a pit where those bodies were, covered in blood. I wanted to get out and couldn't. I was lost.

A veritable nightmare of bodily fragmentation, in which the living are confused with the dead and she falls into the worst of places. Let us note, however, that this is no longer a free fall, but a sliding descent along a slide.

Although I do not mention it, I cannot help associating this experience with her recent visit to her family, where her father constantly speaks of her deceased sister and asserts that C. stands in her place. It will take time for her to distance herself from these statements and from the conflicts that take place there – whether between the father and the mother, between the father and his other children, or the direct aggressions towards her, which are not infrequent on her father's part.

At a certain point, these visits – which C. maintains under the pretext that she works in private households there and saves money for the year – have become more tolerable over time, as she applies with her father the same rule she uses with her sister-in-law: "I don't give it any importance". When she travels to see them, she later tells me about some of her father's aggressions and how, by responding neither yes nor no, she receives fewer affronts and avoids the old, turbulent quarrels.

However, this resource emerges after the dream I am recounting here, one marked by a strong deathly imprint. The long corridors she moves through, the prohibition against passing and the slide that leads her towards death might perhaps have been heard by Freud as a staging of her birth, during which her life was in danger. Yet the dream also informs us of her current state – her *being lost*, her dejection. She will define her post-summer state by saying: "I am shut inside something I cannot define". She finds herself lacking the desire for anything and is doing very little in her day-to-day life.

In the weeks following this dream, I further explore her resources in such moments. It is in this context that the information emerges

about song lyrics and the use she makes of them to come out of certain states. We work in detail on those references that keep her afloat: her favourite singers, her preferred phrases, the times of day at which she chooses to play music.
Shortly thereafter, another dream ensues.

### *9.6.8 Ninth Dream*

> I had a very strange dream. It frightened me. It was a dark place, like a forest [similar to the one near her hometown], and a house resembling one where my mother works. I was there with her and with my brother on my father's side [the one who left when he came of age and never returned]. There was another person who was supposedly his father. He was like a faceless shadow. They had stolen money from me and were running away. I chase them and catch them. They had stolen something that was mine, something I had made myself with all my effort – here she clarifies that it was not known what object had been stolen from her-. I am seized by a moment of fury and I hit him with a stick … until I leave him lifeless. I wasn't able to stop hitting him.

As with the previous one, this dream initially concerns me. As we have seen, although nightmares predominate for her, not all her dreams are so stark and violent. Moreover, I notice a hesitation when she has to state explicitly that she strikes the figure to death; she seems ashamed or uncomfortable. The first thing that occurs to me is to ask her how she has been feeling, and also whether she has noticed in herself anything that might be comparable to that "not being able to stop". Curiously, she reports having felt better that week. The arguments with "this person" have ceased for some time now, and she has not experienced disturbances in other areas of her life. She herself has been taken by surprise by this dream, which she felt a strong urgency to tell me about – to "get it off her chest", one might say. "It frightened me", she says. But then she tells me that she had been reading a book and that she "felt identified". The book stated that people with anxiety disorders are changeable and fearful. This gave her pause for thought, as she is determined to graduate but often encounters obstacles such as drops in her mood, and now she thinks of this as a form of her fear – a fear "of not being able to".

I think that this dream has come to replace the melancholised state in which she had been over the previous weeks. Although it was striking, we should trust her words and thus consider that the dream has taken upon itself the deathly element, thereby freeing for her the possibility of thinking, of subjectivising her fear, and of questioning her capacity to move forward in the course of study she has chosen.

Once the initial impact has passed, I decide to point out something that has stayed with me: that thing of hers, for which there was no need to know what it was. I tell her, then, that it is the first time that this idea has appeared in one of her dreams – of something intimately her own, moreover something gained through her own effort and which no one will be able to take from her. In response to this intervention, I observe a change in C.'s expression; she seems to brighten. It is then that she tells me that she has bought herself a guitar – the first time she has bought something solely for herself.

This dream occurs shortly after I had asked her whether she had considered changing her name – an occasion on which I oppose both her father's version and her own, which positioned her as a mere substitute for her deceased sister. I consider that session to have been the prelude to this dream; and that the intervention which extracts from the account a glimmer of desire – this desire to have something of her own – seems to have been a turning point in C.'s analysis.

Let us also note that this dream takes place after having spoken about her fantasy of motherhood, the one that impacted and moved her so deeply "to the point of tears", as she puts it.

### *9.6.9 Tenth Dream*

A few weeks later, she dreams:

> It was night-time, but not with that same darkness as before. I was in a two-storey house, with a staircase, with unknown people – women. A man had us held captive (myself and two women, one older and one younger). There was mistreatment of every kind, physical, psychological. We could do nothing without his permission. There was also a baby; it belonged to one of the women. At one point he stays with the youngest; there was abuse, rape. We didn't know what to do; we listened from the other room. We protected the baby. He calls us and lines us up. He gives me a shotgun, as if to say that I wouldn't know how to do anything. The

> shotgun fired arrows, not bullets. I shoot at him but miss. I throw the weapon down and run away. The older woman tells me to run and to take the baby. There was a large exit onto the street. The baby was already outside, hidden, covered with a blanket. A voice was saying, 'where is my daughter?'. I run out into the street with the baby in my arms – and that's where I cut it, because I woke up.

Of this dream, so harrowing, I point out that it has an interesting ending. C. agrees. It is an extensive dream – with a narrative plot, many elements and a denouement that is curiously recounted in the first person: "I cut it". In this dream, she leaves and abandons what is torturous within that house. She saves the baby, just as the woman had advised her to do. The baby – herself, Freud would say – was already protected, covered, and out in the street. Here, rather than looking, she listens; she listens from the other room. A shift in the object of the drive.

She fires, but does not hit, does not kill – and this does not prevent her from saving herself.

The account of C.'s treatment ends here. Once the period stipulated by the health service came to an end, she visited me in my private practice on the occasions she considered appropriate.

In the interval during which we make this transition, she passes a final examination that had been preventing her from continuing her studies. She manages this thanks to a friend who offers to explain certain topics to her. That examination, which she had failed twice in previous years, becomes achievable in the encounter with others: with the voice of the friend who explains things to her, with the presence of a fellow student sitting the exam on the same day, and with the virtual encouragement of her friends in the chat. If her studies continue on their course, she will be able to accompany children in the earliest stages of life. Time will tell whether this – or something else – will prove possible for C.

## Notes

1 Note that she has modified the original lyrics, which read: "tu amor es mi enfermedad, soy un envase vacío" ('your love is my illness, I am an empty vessel').

2 Translator's note: "Se me muere" is an idiomatic expression familiar to speakers of Rioplatense Spanish. "It's dying on me" has been chosen as the

closest English equivalent – the "on me" carrying the sense that the dying is happening at the speaker's expense or in their presence, without the speaker being the one who caused it. In English, "it's dying on me" works when referring to an animal but sounds unusual when referring to a person, where the most natural expression would be "he's dying on me" or "she's dying on me". In Spanish, the same expression can refer to a person, an animal, or a thing, without distinguishing between them.

# 10 Working with Dreams as a Clinical Resource

The utility of working with dreams in the analysis of psychotic patients rests on specific technical adjustments and on a firm theoretical appreciation of how the dream functions as a vital mediating space between the subject and the potential irruption of the real. While the traditional reservations regarding the work with dreams in the analysis of psychotics have been noted throughout this book, successful clinical practice calls for alternative strategies and the recognition of the dream's inherent stabilising function.

## 10.1 Beyond Free Association: Precise Questioning and Dream Series

We have mentioned that one of the most frequently cited difficulties in working with psychotic patients is the difficulty of free association. Unlike neurotic patients, who may readily provide further material when questioned about a dream, many psychotic patients struggle to associate freely. This is not, however, an insurmountable obstacle, provided the analyst is willing to supplement the broad invitation of free association with more targeted approaches.

The first of these is to question the dreams with precise inquiries, strictly oriented towards linking dream content to the dreamer's life and subjective position. The value of this approach lies in seeking specific associations that are often difficult for psychotic patients to produce initially.

One productive approach involves paying particular attention to the actions performed in the dream, often expressed through verbs.

DOI: 10.4324/9781003755166-13

Derived from clinical experience and Freudian theory concerning the drives, this approach allows for focused questioning. Let us consider the example of a psychotic analysand's dream reported by De Arriba (2018):

> Begging – that's how I was. I was sleeping on the floor, turning my head from side to side, feeling the burden I carried on my shoulders. I get up with a cane and walk as if I were an old woman with the body of a young one. There were two rows of people, as if it were a church. Then I decided to walk through the middle of those rows. And there were three empresses: one was a young woman, and two were girls, all three dressed in the same way. And the only thing that happened was that we looked at one another. Then I woke up, and afterwards I cried. A strange dream.
>
> (De Arriba, 2018, p.187)

Rather than attempting a broad interpretation of the dream's enigma, the analyst might focus questions on its specific elements and actions. For instance, regarding the verb "to beg": "What relationship do you have with 'begging'? Have you felt as if you were begging in any circumstance?" And regarding the element of the "cane": "What about 'getting up with a cane'? What 'canes' have allowed you to get up at other times in your life? What do you consider your canes to be today, and what are they for?"

This style of questioning attempts to link the dream's statements to the patient's everyday life and their subjective choices, reducing the risk of opening up a "too-broad enigma" that the psychotic patient might then read through the lens of their delusion.

The second approach recognises that, when faced with difficulty in associating with a single dream, the analyst must bear in mind – as we mentioned in Section 8.2 – that dream series can function as genuine associative chains (Boukhabza, 2012, 2013). These series often carry greater informational value than a single dream. Referred to as *continued stories* by Freud, subsequent dreams may arise in response to the questions posed or left open by prior ones. Through this process, a central theme can be progressively elaborated, often at a pace that exceeds what the psychotic consciously registers. If the analyst sustains the transferential focus on the dreams, the patient can attend to material emerging from their unconscious – material they might otherwise be unable to access through consciousness.

## 10.2 Dreams as an Effective Remedy Against the Return in the Real

The most significant theoretical and clinical consequence of working with dreams in psychoses is that the dream can constitute an effective remedy against the return in the real. This claim rests on a fundamental distinction between symptoms returning in the real – such as unmediated hallucinations or delusional certainties – and the process of oneiric elaboration.

The dream scene, understood as the Other scene constitutive of the unconscious, allows for the displacement of elements derived from the delusion or hallucination onto the dream's metaphorical and symbolic stage, enabling the subject to recognise them as their own and to work through them differently.

Dream-work may be said to accomplish at least three important functions in this regard. First, it puts ineffable experiences into discourse: dreams collaborate in verbalising the otherwise ineffable experiences of the psychotic's past or present, gathering and giving form to a whole series of suppressed thoughts that might otherwise remain inarticulate in waking life. This allows the analyst to intervene opportunely on phenomena – such as initial hallucinatory experiences or emerging delusional ideas – that are currently taking shape. Second, it facilitates historisation: dreams allow for a reconstruction of the subject's experience, recalling initial hallucinatory experiences or moments of estrangement – such as those experienced by the Wolf Man in relation to the walnut-tree – and inserting isolated signifiers, which previously returned via hallucination or delusion, into a new, historisable narrative framework. Third, it represents pathological ideas; thus, dream interpretation provides a means to distil the underlying pathological idea – whether a hysterical fantasy, an obsessional representation, or a delusion – upon which the dream was constructed. This process progressively calls into question the certainty provided by the delusion, leading to the construction of a new subjective history that serves as a fresh point of support for life.

When a patient, having gained some distance from the initial certainty of their delusion, accepts some questioning of their subjective choices, their dreams will collaborate in revealing the subjective position commanding their repetition. The signifiers of the dream, directed towards the analyst and recognised with surprise by the patient as part of their own unconscious, may progressively call into question the delusion that previously maintained the subject's submission to the *jouissance* of the Other. Dream-work, like the analytic process itself, thus makes use of the unconscious to allow the subject to advance in their know-how regarding their symptom.

## 10.3 Dreams as Indicators of the Direction of the Treatment

Once the transference is properly established, dreams often provide important indications for the direction of the treatment – conveying operations that need to be produced in the treatment. These are singular to each case and may include: producing a new knowledge to replace the knowledge offered by the voices; effecting a necessary separation from the Other; accompanying the formation of a new life following subjective devastation; or embodying a vital brake on infinite metonymy.

One significant direction that dreams can convey concerns the very operation the analyst must perform within the session. In one clinical case communicated under supervision many years ago, a psychotic analysand dreamed of a train moving at full speed until a person, facing it with their hand raised, brought it to a halt. When the analyst enquired about the dream, the patient began to engage in endless, senseless associations – an infinite metonymy. The analyst, feeling disorientated, reacted by halting the discourse and making a sharp cut to the associative chain. Here, the dream of the train that needed to be stopped was not only staged in the session itself but also served as a probable reference to the function expected of the analyst in that particular treatment: embodying a vital brake on infinite metonymy.

Dreams can also indicate a progression in the subjective position that needs to be achieved through the analytic act. In another example, a psychotic patient recounted two dreams. In the first, she was being observed from a window; in the second, she was the one observing, with other people *interposed* between her and the person being observed. The second dream demonstrated a clear progression regarding the subject's relationship to observation and the Other's gaze, indicating the necessary direction of the treatment.

Even when the psychotic patient firmly rejects the content of their dream or refuses to associate, the dream still provides the analyst with crucial information about the patient's subjective position, which can be used with care in subsequent interventions. Dreams thus convey the operations that need to be produced in each singular treatment – making them, as we have argued throughout this book, an indispensable resource in the analytic work with psychoses.

# Final Remarks

We have reviewed Freud's developments concerning the specific mechanism that allows the psychotic to repress a thought through projection. We have also seen that what is repressed in this way coexists with a partial recognition of that which has been rejected. We were able to observe that, in C., the sorrow of having been positioned as a usurper of the name and the life of her deceased sister coexists with the projection by which she makes of her sister-in-law a usurper, worthy of fear and hatred. A certain rectification of her position begins with a dream in which she is confronted with her role in the disorder that arose between herself, her brother, and her sister-in-law; yet this rectification is, at that moment, decidedly rejected. Later on, however – and as if the dream had struck home – C. progressively adopts a position that allows her not to initiate arguments and thus to suffer less in cohabitation. But we must not overlook that this rectification coexists with the certainty, preserved intact, that her sister-in-law, "this person", is a usurper – a jouissant Other from whom it is advisable for her to keep her distance.

This allows us to say that the dream has introduced into C.'s analysis a partial rectification, the value of which should not be underestimated, as it entails significant changes in her everyday life and in her economy of *jouissance.*

What we find particularly compelling in this trajectory – across the question of dreams in psychoses – is that of effects at the level of the unconscious which do not entail a passage through consciousness. We believe that this matter has already been extensively considered in relation to the analysis of neurotics, and it is the central point addressed by Lacan in *The Error of the Subject Supposed to Know*

(1967), where he defends the idea that analysts very often forget that the unconscious, in the strict sense, neither passes nor will ever pass through consciousness.

We have the clinical impression that, in psychotic subjects, this fact is even more clear-cut, since we observe that in analyses, even when there is work with the unconscious, some psychotic analysands are not adept at associating – a well-known fact, and one which should not be forgotten, since it also implies the necessary participation of consciousness – and they remain in a position of not knowing that which their own unconscious produces. If we were to remain with this observation, however, we would be overlooking the very noticeable effects produced by that same work, for the participation of consciousness does not appear to be the key for those effects to occur.

The analysis of psychotics thus shows us, with greater clarity, something that we ought to bear more firmly in mind in neurotic cases: that the participation of consciousness is merely secondary; that the effects of working with ciphered material exceed the reach of conscious thought and are manifested above all in libidinal modifications. The psychotic's rejection of what their unconscious returns to them is here the most compelling proof of this fact, and we believe it should neither intimidate analysts nor discourage them from working with such material. As Boukhabza maintains, even if the psychotic can scarcely associate at all, they will bring other dreams, subsequent ones, which will serve as associations for what could not be said at that moment. And in this unfolding, the analyst will apprehend the effects taking place in the analysand's everyday life – a subject who, despite not seeming to take notice of their own productions, has indeed done so, and in a most dignified manner.

# References


American Psychiatric Association (APA). (1994). *Manual Diagnóstico y Estadístico de los Trastornos Mentales DSM-IV-TR*. Masson.

Apollon, W. (2008a) La logique de la cure du psychotique. En W. Apollon, D. Bergeron y L. Cantin, *La cure psychanalytique du psychotique. Enjeux et stratégies* (pp. 47–86). Gifric.

Apollon, W. (2008b) Métapsychologie et clinique dans le traitement psychanalytique des psychoses. En W. Apollon, D. Bergeron y L. Cantin, *La cure psychanalytique du psychotique. Enjeux et stratégies* (pp. 21–46). Gifric.

Bergeron, D. (2008) Le corps au rythme de la cure analytique du psychotique. En W. Apollon, D. Bergeron y L. Cantin, *La cure psychanalytique du psychotique. Enjeux et stratégies* (pp. 217–260). Gifric.

Boukhabza, D. (2012) *La lettre du rêve. Un lecteur pour la psychose*. Érès.

Boukhabza, D. (2013) Le rêve, un outil pour la cure analytique des psychoses. *Psychologie Clinique, 36*, 184–192.

Cantin, L. (2008) Avènement de la parole, déconstruction du délire et expérience de «castration» dans la cure du psychotique. En W. Apollon, D. Bergeron y L. Cantin, *La cure psychanalytique du psychotique. Enjeux et stratégies* (pp. 173–216). Gifric.

Capozzi, P.; De Masi, F. (2001) The Meaning of Dreams in the Psychotic State. *International Journal of Psychoanalysis, 82*, 933–952.

De Arriba, J. P. (2018) *Los sueños en las psicosis*. Letra Viva.

De Battista, J. (2015) *El deseo en las psicosis*. Letra Viva.

Escars, C. J. (2002) *Los nombres de los lobos. Lecturas de un caso célebre*. Imago Mundi.

Freud, S. (1894/1981a) The Neuro-Psychoses of Defence. In *The Standard Edition of the Complete Psychological Works of Sigmund Freud* (Vol. 3). The Hogarth Press.

Freud, S. (1896/1999) Nuevas puntualizaciones sobre las neuropsicosis de defensa. *En Obras Completas* (J. L. Etcheverry, trad., Vol. 3). Amorrortu.

Freud, S. (1900/1971) The Interpretation of Dreams (First Part). In *The Standard Edition of the Complete Psychological Works of Sigmund Freud* (Vol. 4 & 5). The Hogarth Press.

Freud, S. (1901/2001) Psicopatología de la vida cotidiana. En *Obras Completas* (J. L. Etcheverry, trad., Vol. 6). Amorrortu.

Freud, S. (1911/1981) Psycho-Analytic Notes on an Autobiographical Account of a Case of Paranoia (Dementia Paranoides). In *The Standard Edition of the Complete Psychological Works of Sigmund Freud* (Vol. 12). The Hogarth Press.

Freud, S. (1913/2000) Tótem y tabú. Algunas concordancias en la vida anímica de los salvajes y de los neuróticos. En Amorrortu, *Obras Completas* (J. L. Etcheverry, trad., Vol. 13). Amorrortu.

Freud, S. (1915/2000a) La represión. En Amorrortu, *Obras Completas* (J. L. Etcheverry, trad., Vol. 14). Amorrortu.

Freud, S. (1915/2000b) Lo inconsciente. En Amorrortu, *Obras Completas* (J. L. Etcheverry, trad., Vol. 14). Amorrortu.

Freud, S. (1918/1999) De la historia de una neurosis infantil. En Amorrortu, *Obras Completas* (J. L. Etcheverry, trad., Vol. 17). Amorrortu.

Freud, S. (1919/1981) The 'Uncanny'. In *The Standard Edition of the Complete Psychological Works of Sigmund Freud* (Vol. 17). The Hogarth Press.

Freud, S. (1922/1981) Some Neurotic Mechanisms in Jealousy, Paranoia and Homosexuality. In *The Standard Edition of the Complete Psychological Works of Sigmund Freud* (Vol. 18). The Hogarth Press.

Freud, S. (1923/1981) Remarks on the Theory and Practice of Dream-Interpretation. In *The Standard Edition of the Complete Psychological Works of Sigmund Freud* (Vol. 19). The Hogarth Press.

Freud, S. (1933/1981) Revision of the Theory of Dreams. In *The Standard Edition of the Complete Psychological Works of Sigmund Freud* (Vol. 22). The Hogarth Press.

Kolko, C. (2004) *Les absents de la mémoire*. Érès.

Labaronnie, C. (2016) Algunas contribuciones sobre los sueños de fin de análisis. *Anuario de Investigaciones, 23,* 101–107.

Labaronnie, C.; Lombardi, G. (2018) Algunas posiciones subjetivas frente a lo pulsional en los sueños. *Revista Latinoamericana de Psicopatologia Fundamental, São Paulo, 21(1),* 58–80.

Lacan, J. (1932) *La psicosis paranoica*. Recuperado de www.lacanterafreudiana.com.ar/2.5.1.1%20%20%20-LAPSICOSIS%20PARANOICA.%20TESIS%20DOCTORADO%20LACAN,%201932.pdf

Lacan, J. (1946/1985): "Acerca de la causalidad psíquica". *En Escritos 1* (pp. 142–183). Bs. As., Siglo XXI Editores.

Lacan, J. (1955–56/1997) The Psychoses. In *The Seminar of Jacques Lacan (Book 3)*, Translated by Russell Grigg. Norton.

Lacan, J. (1957/2003) El psicoanálisis y su enseñanza. En *Escritos 1* (pp. 419–440). Siglo XXI.

Lacan, J. (1959/2005) De una cuestión preliminar a todo tratamiento posible de la psicosis. En Siglo XXI, *Escritos 2* (pp. 513–564). Siglo XXI.

Lacan, J. (1960–61/2009). La transferencia. En *El seminario* (libro 8). Buenos Aires: Paidós.

Lacan, J. (1962–63/2006) La angustia. En *El seminario* (libro 10). Paidós.

Lacan, J. (1967/2012) La equivocación del sujeto supuesto saber. En Paidós, *Otros Escritos*. Paidós.

Lacan, J. (1970) *Radiophonie*. Online version, translated by J. W. Stone's. www.lacantokyo.org/img/Radiophonie_tr_en.pdf

Lacan, J. (1972) *Conferencia en Lovaina*. Recuperado de www.lacanterafreudiana.com.ar/2.5.1.21%20%20%20%20CONFERENCIA%20EN%20LOVAINA,%201972.pdf

Lacan, J. (1973/2012). Televisón. En Paidós, *Otros escritos* (pp. 535–572). Paidós.

Lacan, J. (1975/2007) *La Troisième*. Online version, Translated by Y. Szczech. www.researchgate.net/publication/307210365_Lacan's_La_Troisieme_English_Translation

Lacan, J. (1975–76/2016) The Sinthome. In *The Seminar of Jacques Lacan (Book 23)*. Polity Press.

Lacan, J. (1977–78) Le moment de conclure. En *Le séminaire* (libro 25). Inédito. Recuperado de http://staferla.free.fr/S25/S25.htm

Lombardi, G. (2015) *La libertad en psicoanálisis*. Paidós.

Lombardi, G. (2018, septiembre) *El discurso analítico, garante de la histerización del analizante*. Ponencia presentada en el VI Encuentro Internacional de Escuela de Psicoanálisis de los Foros del Campo Lacaniano, Barcelona. Inédito.

Lombardi, G.; Laje, M. (2016) La culpa como índice de la posición del sujeto en el deseo. *Anuario de investigaciones, 23*, 109–116.

Mazzuca, M. (2011) *Ecos del pase*. Letra Viva.

Paola, D. (1994) *Psicosis o cuerpo*. Laderiva.

Sauvagnat, F. & Sauvagnat, R. (1998) Fenómenos elementales y estabilizaciones en las psicosis maníaco-depresivas. *Revista de la Asociación Española de Neuropsiquiatría, 18(67)*, pp. 459–470. Recuperado de www.documentacion.aen.es/pdf/revista-aen/1998/revista-67/04-fenomenos_elementales_y_estabilizadores.pdf

Schreber, D. P. (1903/2000) *Memoirs of My Nervous Illness*. Harvard University Press.

Soler, C. (2004/2007) El rechazo del inconsciente. En *¿Qué se espera del psicoanálisis y del psicoanalista? Conferencias y seminarios en Argentina* (pp. 239–251). Letra Viva.

Vetere, E. (2014) *La invención psicótica de la transferencia.* En Lazos. Lazos.

Yacoi, A. (2002) Sueños en la conclusión de los análisis. *Mediodichos.*

Yacoi, A. (2012) Sueño y fin de análisis, una introducción. En L. Ávola, A. Cucagna y A. Yacoi, *Brisas clínicas: sueño y final de análisis* (pp. 129–133). Grama.

# Index

For Product Safety Concerns and Information please contact our EU representative GPSR@taylorandfrancis.com
Taylor & Francis Verlag GmbH, Kaufingerstraße 24, 80331 München, Germany

www.ingramcontent.com/pod-product-compliance
Ingram Content Group UK Ltd.
Pitfield, Milton Keynes, MK11 3LW, UK
UKHW021953220926
475880UK00003B/22

* 9 7 8 1 0 4 1 2 7 5 8 7 9 *